# THROUGH WINDOWS
# OF OPPORTUNITY

# THROUGH WINDOWS
# OF OPPORTUNITY

## A Neuroaffective Approach
## to Child Psychotherapy

*Marianne Bentzen and Susan Hart*

**KARNAC**

First published in Danish in 2013 as *Jagten på de nonspecifikke faktorer i psykoterapi med børn* by
Hans Reitzels Forlag, Copenhagen


First published in English in 2015 by
Karnac Books Ltd
118 Finchley Road, London NW3 5HT

British Library Cataloguing in Publication Data

A C.I.P. for this book is available from the British Library

ISBN 978 1 78220 158 8

Edited, designed and produced by The Studio Publishing Services Ltd
www.publishingservicesuk.co.uk
e-mail: studio@publishingservicesuk.co.uk

Printed in Great Britain


www.karnacbooks.com

# CONTENTS

# ABOUT THE AUTHORS

**Marianne Bentzen** is a neuroaffective psychotherapist. She has been leading professional trainings in somatic psychotherapy in Europe and North America since 1982. Her focus today is on the practical applications of neuroaffective developmental psychology, PTSD treatment, mindfulness practice, and systemic processes. She has authored numerous articles for professional publications in Danish, English, and German.

**Susan Hart** is a psychologist, who is a specialist and supervisor in child psychology and in psychotherapy. With a background in family treatment and child psychiatry, Susan is now in private practice. In her extensive lecture and workshop activity, she develops and teaches the neuroaffective concept developed from recent brain research. She has written ten other books on the subject of neuroaffective developmental psychology and psychotherapy, of which two are published in English.

## Colwyn Trevarthen

Human sense is understanding how to live in the human and physical worlds that children normally develop in the first few years of life. It is learned spontaneously in direct encounters with these worlds that arise unavoidably everywhere, transcending cultural differences. The learning is always informed and guided by emotion – that is, by feelings of significance, of value, of what matters. And it is highly stable and enduring, once established. It is the foundation on which all that follows must build.

> (Margaret Donaldson, personal communication.
> See her book, *Children's Minds*, 1978, on the
> motives of human sense and school learning)

### Supporting the natural spirit of the child, and its growth in companionship

In every human community, whatever its culture, from the most "communal" to the most "private", from the smallest and least technical to the global and most advanced in artificial ways of collaborative life, parents and grandparents delight in the vitality and creativity of their children. They value how a young human being brings a love of affectionate company and enjoyment of adventurous play. The youngest of infants do not only sleep, or make strident calls for care and comfort of the body. They act with purposeful co-ordination of their organs of movement and sensation, showing interest and affective judgement. In intimate encounters, they smile and imitate many expressions with emotions of interest and enjoyment (Kugiumutzakis & Trevarthen, 2014), and they soon take active part in the composition of imaginative conversations, action games, and songs (Trevarthen, 1986, 2006; Trevarthen & Delafield-Butt, 2013). The rhythmic stories of baby songs have the same timings as action games involving shared movements of the hands and body. They can be dance or song, and often are both together (Eckerdal & Merker, 2009). In the Kalahari desert, Takada (2005) has studied how mothers of the !Xun people exercise the playful young bodies of their infants aged about six months, when they can just stand, by bouncing them in "baby gymnastics", which prepares them for later dancing with other children. We learn essential values of life from accepting and accompanying this innate human spirit of moving and its conviviality, and feel we must protect it from harm and help when it is distressed.

We need also to recognise that the active process of growth and learning has a programme not only for the immediate or proximal future, but for more distant times that make up steps of a lifetime. Age-related stages mark development of the body with development of the brain, and the changes affect the motives to regulate the functions of the body, to engage with and perceive the world, and to relate to people, including parents, siblings, and teachers or therapists (Trevarthen & Aitken, 2003). The young person—infant, toddler, school child, adolescent, or adult—is changing in impulses to share meanings and feelings of life in a community.

This book brings the expertise of four child psychotherapists together for a wide-ranging and penetrating discussion of the factors that affect early development of relationships and understanding in actual therapeutic encounters which they examined together by micro-analysis of videos recording their work. They use different sciences and different metaphors to characterise their methods of therapy with children and their parents and family, but all use videos to teach their method of working with children, and all recognise the importance of the subtle micro-moments of change in the present, and the shared "composition" of narratives of feeling and recollecting. Peter Levine is an expert on motor defence mechanisms of the body and regulation of bodily feelings of safety and risk by the autonomic system. Jukka Mäkelä applies the performance of Theraplay engagements with the child to establish trust in risk-taking games and active, rhythmic story-making. Haldor Øvreeide uses developmentally supportive dialogue and self-organising in relationships in the "lived moment". Eia Asen, working in London, employs "multi-family therapy" and "mentalization-based family therapy" to support shared rational examination of anxieties and emotional factors that limit awareness and imagination.

Together, under the supportive guidance of Marianne Bentzen and Susan Hart, these four presented and discussed their work in a two-day conference in Copenhagen on "The quest for the non-specific factors in psychotherapy with children", which was transcribed, leading to a book in Danish of which this volume is the English translation.

While they bring different interests and knowledge to bear on their work, and to interpret the recordings, all agreed that support for healthy development, or encouragement of recovery of it after severe distress or neglect, needs to engage with the child's own experience, in the present, in ways that must seek to release the latent force for growth in self-confidence and satisfaction. All considered their work to be in alliance with parents and others who share the child's life. The child therapist is a guide and companion for all these, not an expert instructing them.

Sometimes, children are sad and withdrawn, or angry and defiant. Their anticipation of taking pleasure by being alive with trusted companions in a kind and joyful world is too strong. It can sense betrayal and will fight against misfortune, as well as cry out in pain. Maltreatment or neglect corrupts the plan for development of skills for relating (Perry, 2002; Trevarthen et al., 2006). To help, we have to find ways that will "follow the child" in order to restore the natural creative optimism and sense of fun. To do that effectively, a parent, teacher, or therapist has to recall and appreciate, not just the fragility and dependence of childhood, but especially its will to find both security in the body and joy by living with communal invention—to be well and to play with ways of moving that others will want to share, for fun.

The latest science of human "mirroring" of actions and awareness for self and with others is seeking to recover this understanding of the integrated self and its time-regulated purposes, and ways in which the acting human person relates with others (Ammaniti & Gallese, 2014; Goodrich, 2010). Correlations of prefrontal cortex activity with processes of rational representation and explanation need to be put in affective context. As Haldor Øvreeide says, "If we as therapists cannot use words in a way that links experiences with symbols, we will have words that are not words; they are dead words. And we have societies that are full of dead words. A word without emotion is not a word. It does not connect."

Seeking to find secure common ground for their adventurous work in neuroaffective developmental psychology, the authors accepted the model of Paul MacLean's triune brain to describe the three levels of function of the deep autonomic nervous system, the intermediate limbic system, and the superior prefrontal "mentalizing" system. Conceiving these as a hierarchy of "compasses" that might guide impulses and feelings of expressive behaviour, they further devised a map of the territory to be explored for each system with orthogonal co-ordinates, or axes, of "arousal regulation" (active or sympathetic and passive or parasympathetic) and "hedonic tone" (pleasure *vs.* displeasure) for the autonomic compass, of positive and negative emotional valence across "altercentric participation" *vs.* "egocentric participation" for the limbic compass, and high and low "reflective functioning" with activation or inhibition of "impulse" to take action for the prefrontal compass of "volitional regulation". Each compass has four quadrants in which interactions of the self with any other, including the therapist, are acted out.

These mappings culminated in a triangulation that allowed four contributors to the discussion of their methods to summarise the communications regulated between the child, a parent, and the therapist, in which the therapist aims to optimise the relationship between the child and the parent. In conclusion, special emphasis was placed on the importance of considering the child's capacity, with its family, to live in the community and to make good relationships there.

I am a biologist who has spent most of my academic life as a researcher and teacher of early child development, using descriptive methods with the aid of micro-analysis of film, video, and audio recordings. I have also long been interested in the advancing knowledge of the creative development of the brain and its function in guiding the agency, awareness, and well-being of the body. How movements of intended action and of self-regulation become messages for other human minds is a core preoccupation. I have no experience of child therapy, but the practical message of this book convinces me that the neuroaffective approach to the support and guidance of a child's capacities and opportunities for development gives precious information about how brain and body serve the young mind and regulate how it shares meaning with other minds. The findings and detailed evidence from case studies of "magic and transformation", so carefully presented and interpreted, will be of great value, not only for child therapists and those whom they train, but for all teachers and students of developmental psychology as well. It has important information for neurophysiology and both affective and cognitive neuroscience, too.

# Introduction

Many efficacy studies of therapy have proven that successful thera-peutic processes depend much more on the therapist's ability to main-tain a close personal presence with the client than it does on method and theory. For example, Orlinsky and Howard (1986) found that clients who trusted their therapist were far more co-operative and able to attune. This finding led to a growing interest in so-called non-specific factors (Wampold, 2001). Although practitioners of various therapeutic methods like to emphasise their unique differences, the therapeutic relationship is probably the single most powerful and curative factor, and there are far more similarities than differences in therapists' actual interactions with their clients in any successful therapeutic process. Psychotherapy essentially revolves around a fundamental human need to feel seen and understood by another person, a need that stems in evolutionary terms from the mammal's need to develop social bonds with others.

Among other achievements, modern developmental psychology, with Louis Sander, Ed Tronick, Colwyn Trevarthen, and Daniel Stern among its leading proponents, has identified how microscopic synchronisation processes in the interaction result in profound personality changes, whether they unfold in the healthy carer–child relationship or in the psychotherapeutic process. It is the reciprocal emotional attunement between therapist and child that mediates the treatment, and the only intervention capable of healing inadequate attachment is the establishment of an attachment that is based on adaptive emotional attunement.

These insights inspired us to explore the transformation processes that might escape the therapist's perception. All good therapists have a method that helps them know how to proceed, but it is not the method that produces the essential profound personality-transforming processes. The method indicates a systematic use of certain "tools" and provides a structure for macro-regulation. It consists of the specific tools and principles that are needed to generate transformation processes, comparable to the process of composing music. The rhythm, tempo, and interactive sensitivity of the micro-regulations in the session can be compared to the recurring and unfolding themes in music, and, just as in music, sudden openings appear, leading to new experiences of meaningful states of self-experience. The micro-regulation processes that occur in this musical process stimulate the brain's emotional structures and generate development.

About two decades ago, the Boston Change Study Group was formed, with Daniel Stern, Louis Sander, and Ed Tronick among its leading members. The group explored the present moments in psychotherapy, the brief moments of meeting in psychotherapy where change processes take place. In his later book *The Present Moment in Psychotherapy and Everyday Life* (2004), Daniel Stern offered a definition of present moment. The work and findings of the Boston Change Study Group inspired us to pursue the question of how these moments of change appear in practice.

In recent years, we have actively explored how neuroaffective developmental psychology can be translated into neuroaffective psychotherapy (for more information about our neuroaffective work, visit our website: neuroaffect.eu). On this journey of discovery, it has become increasingly clear to us that emotional development is driven by subtle micro-regulation processes in interpersonal interactions, and that salient interactions must take place in the zone of proximal development. This stimulates the neural areas that will eventually develop the individuals' capacity for mentalization. We live in an age when psychotherapeutic approaches compete for recognition as the most evidence-based and effective method. When a particular psychotherapeutic method is presented, the presenter typically describes the framework and, in many cases, the psychotherapeutic context, as well as the expected macro-regulation processes. In part, this is because the universal micro-regulation processes that mediate the actual development process are extremely difficult to describe, and they can also be exceedingly difficult to observe. Since child therapy is currently undergoing tremendous development, we wanted to create a professional context that explored these micro-regulatory present moments in family and child therapy. Accordingly, we decided to bring together four practitioners who are, in our opinion, among the world's leading psychotherapists in the field of child and family therapy. Their therapeutic methods are very different, but they base their teaching on the same approach, which is to show a video clip of a therapy session with a child.

On 19 and 20 June 2012 in Copenhagen, these representatives of four different psychotherapy methods met in person: Peter Levine from the USA represented somatic experiencing, Jukka Mäkelä from Finland represented the Theraplay approach, Haldor Øvreeide from Norway introduced developmentally supportive dialogues with children and parents, and Eia Asen from the UK presented a multi-family mentalization-based framework. We shared these historic and unforgettable days with some 240 enthusiastic and interested participants. The conference was titled "The quest for the non-specific factors in psychotherapy with children". After the event, we received overwhelmingly positive feedback from conference participants who were keen to share their enthusiasm with us, and the Danish book about the event, published in September 2013, has been greeted with the same immense enthusiasm. It is with great pleasure that we now share our own excitement about this exploration with a wider audience.

At the conference, we asked the four therapists to share and discuss the factors common to their psychotherapeutic interventions with children rather than focusing on the factors that differentiate their individual methods. We asked each of them to show a video clip of themselves interacting with a child in a therapeutic context and to explain what they thought was important in the micro-regulation process, *without* focusing on the method or the macro-regulation. After each therapist's presentation, we asked them to share their thoughts about the moments of change they noticed in the video excerpt and the reflections it sparked. Thus, the two-day event aimed to examine and identify the common human potential for creating psychological transformation processes, including interpersonal as well as, ultimately, intrapsychic change.

We felt that bringing together this unique group of psychothera- pists marked a historic event, and, therefore, we arranged with the Danish publishing house, Hans Reitzels, to have a representative in place to transcribe everything that was said during the two-day con- ference. In return, we promised to use the transcript as the basis for a book that would allow a much larger audience than the conference participants to benefit from the meeting.

At the conference, we first introduced the neuroaffective com- passes that are discussed in Chapters Two to Six of this book to provide a framework and offer a general theory, or "map", that might act as a shared navigational instrument and help us understand the present moments from the perspective of neuroaffective develop- mental psychology. These compasses reflect some of the most impor- tant developmental challenges that the infant faces in the earliest development and maturation of the brain, as it transitions from a *sensing* to an *emotional* and, eventually, a *mentalizing* and fully devel- oped human brain. We discussed the three compasses in relation to key intrapsychological states that unfold on these three levels and which can be described in relation to an autonomic sensory, a limbic emotional, and a prefrontal mentalizing compass. The compasses provided a rich framework for describing both the ideal course of development and the very real risk of the child being thrown off course developmentally, and for discussing how even our adult lives can be plagued by acquired imbalances, which the compasses can help us understand. Our presentation of the compasses in their devel- opmental sequence also determined the sequence of the four very different presentations, videos, and psychotherapeutic methods. In their presentations, the four therapists described their interventions and shared some of the effective moments in their psychotherapies with the audience. Peter Levine was the first presenter, followed by Jukka Mäkelä, Haldor Øvreeide, and, finally, Eia Asen. They all demonstrated very convincingly that it is possible to re-establish a secure attachment or to overcome a trauma, through moments of presence and contact, when the meeting is established on the right level and in an attachment relationship.

The conference programme moved from the bottom up, beginning with a look at the brain's earliest maturing structures, the autonomic nervous system. Peter Levine has developed the method "somatic experiencing", which operates on a bodily level to meet and dissolve the inhibition of instinctive defence mechanisms that have emerged during life-threatening events. In a review of two therapy videos, Peter Levine demonstrated how he focuses on arousal waves and bodily contact rhythms to allow incomplete motor defensive responses from the original threatening event to be expressed. In this process, he ensures that the child is not overwhelmed, but is, in fact, able to integrate and reorganise his or her joy-filled interaction capacity, resulting in improved self-regulation in the autonomic nervous system.

In the afternoon, we discussed the mid-brain structures that make up the limbic system, and which mediate early attachment. Jukka Mäkelä, a Finnish child psychiatrist and child psychotherapist trained in Theraplay in Chicago, used video clips to demonstrate the potentials of Theraplay to reorganise and rebuild insecure attachment patterns. In Theraplay, the therapist uses an active, intensely contact-building and profoundly appreciative interaction that helps the child overcome the emotional difficulties resulting from severe attachment disorders. The method relies on sensitive and organising touch, rough-and-tumble play with the adult, and joy-filled interactions.

On the second day of the conference, we first met the Norwegian psychologist Haldor Øvreeide, who has developed the developmentally supportive dialogue, which assumes that the child is born with predispositions for recognising others and for finding, responding to, and adapting to "the other". In the developmentally supportive dialogue, children are motivated to express themselves in their own terms within an adaptive framework that lets them bring their subjective perspective forward, and which respects their self-organisation. From a neuroaffective compass perspective, this facilitates the child's development of prefrontal self-narratives.

The conference was concluded with a video review of a family therapy process carried out by Eia Asen. Eia Asen is a child psychiatrist and has developed multi-family therapy (MFT) and mentalization-based family therapy (MBFT); until 2013, he was the clinical director of the Marlborough Family Service in London and he now works at the Anna Freud Centre. He described the goal of mentalization-based family therapy as uncovering dysfunctional patterns in the

family members' mutual interaction and communication and to experiment with new and more functional patterns that may then, in turn,
become objects for reflection. Asen emphasises relational observations
over individual observations and argues that altering the context will
require the child as well as the parents to mentalize. In his work, he
further supports the development of the prefrontal mentalization
capacity with numerous questions, often about the child's or the
parent's respective perception of the other's experience or about their
current understanding of earlier events in the course of therapy.

As we set out with the basic assumption that the therapeutic
approaches presented were not in conflict with one another, but
instead addressed different levels of the child's development, the
panel debates focused on uncovering the non-specific factors in the
various interventions. In the course of the conference, it soon became
clear that one universal condition for effective present moments in
psychotherapy is that the child and the parents feel heard and seen.
Another condition is that the meeting has a relevant and curative aim,
as the therapist brings his or her knowledge and experience to bear in
an effort to improve the respective capacities and conditions of the
child and the parents

The purpose of the conference was to home in on the present
moments in psychotherapy and to define them in even more detail
than the Boston Change Study Group had done. All the presented
methods had emerged and developed in the context of clinical practice,
and a core element in them all was the belief in the inherent wisdom of
how interacting human systems offer essential information for growth,
presented by the child in each "unfolding present moment".

Haldor Øvreeide explained that if the psychotherapist is able to
capture the present moment and reflect it back to the child and the
parents, the unfolding moment becomes a "lived moment", which is
witnessed, shared, and realised with the significant other that the
therapist temporarily represents. As Øvreeide pointed out, psychotherapy with children initially unfolds in a relationship with asymmetrical responsibility, where the therapist always has a specific goal
and intention with the therapy, as well as the responsibility for
framing the process. However, within this framework, the process
unfolds in a symmetrical and shared exploration of the child's and the
parents' current problem, which they resolve themselves through
their own discoveries.

Eia Asen takes a more radical approach: "If people have an eating problem I want to see how they eat; if people have a sleeping problem I want to see how they sleep; and if they've got a toilet problem we want to know how that works . . ." Although the latter comment was tongue-in-cheek, it illustrates the underlying premise of the clinic's work, which is to maintain the family setting while introducing challenges and questions as the child and parents engage in their own process of discovery in relation to the issues and come up with creative and unpredictable solutions.

Jukka Mäkelä and Peter Levine both expressed similar points of view, although their approaches address more archaic brain structures and meetings and stage activities that get in "under the child's and the parents' radar", to quote Peter Levine. Both Mäkelä's and Levine's interventions are more experiential and preverbal in nature. More primitive brain structures and impulses are met on their own terms, and the psychotherapist offers a context to help the organism unfold its own creative solutions to the unmet developmental challenges.

In closing, the four therapists reflected on the similarities between the therapist and the archetype of "the magical stranger": like Mary Poppins, the therapist arrives in a situation to address an arrested development process, utilising novel interactions that emphasise motor impulses, emotions, imagination, playfulness, and creativity. As Jukka Mäkelä pointed out, there is obviously no single approach that always works, and no single therapy form is always effective. Perhaps the therapist simply is not capable enough, or perhaps the parent, for a variety of reasons, is unable to transfer the process back to the family life, making it difficult for the child to change.

Thus, the conference sought to identify some of the specific factors that cross methodological boundaries and give rise to the present moments in psychotherapy. At the conference, the concept of "windows of opportunity" was mentioned repeatedly. We also returned repeatedly to reflections on the zone of proximal development, phrased in the general question, "What works for whom?" The presenters agreed that there is always an open window somewhere for the children, the parents, and the therapists to discover. There is always an opportunity, and if we fail to grasp a present moment, another will come. The therapist should never lose heart, and, as Haldor Øvreeide pointed out, we can always become better at offering children developmental possibilities. We can always learn more about what types of elements or qualities are required to enable these developmental moments, but it is always the child's response that determines whether any given moment becomes a developmental moment. As psychotherapists, we must remain open to spontaneous occurrences, because change is always spontaneous. If we were to try to control the spontaneous process, we would, in fact, prevent the developmental moment from occurring.

With their individual approaches, the four therapists are all pursuing what should be a human right: to re-establish the natural experience of being met with love, understanding, and care, on the appropriate level, whether after a life-threatening experience or after the denial of the right to love, intimacy, attachment, and appreciation. Each in their way, the four presenters based their actual interventions on meeting children where they are and allowing them to develop their inherent potential within a loving, gentle, and attachment-related perspective.

As a result of millions of years of evolution, the human brain is now "designed" to synchronise with other human autonomic nervous systems, attune affectively with other human limbic systems, and interpret our own and others' intentions through its prefrontal structures. A mature personality structure that engages with others through compassion, empathy, and reflection initially develops in interaction with close attachment figures. To reach our full personality potential, we need stimulation: we need to be synchronised, mirrored, and contained in interactions with other people, as this develops the brain's emotional and personality potential. If this process has failed to unfold adequately during the developmental "windows of opportunity", the child needs targeted support to develop his or her emotional structures. In other words, the child needs a "fairy godmother" who can enter the child's life for a time to support both the child's and the parents' developmental process.

It was very rewarding to see the rich video material from the four psychotherapists at the conference, and we have tried to describe and represent them as clearly and loyally as possible in writing. We would like to take this opportunity to thank the children and parents in the videos for their permission to use the material in a written form and for their contribution to clarify the profound micro-regulating processes in child psychotherapy. These recordings and their written documentation are an invaluable source of learning. To preserve the anonymity of the children and parents involved, we have altered their names in the descriptions, although the children's real names were used at the conference.

## An overview of the book

As described, the book is based on the two-day conference "The quest for the non-specific factors in psychotherapy with children", and, unless otherwise indicated, all the quotes in the book and all the epigraphs to the chapters are from the conference. Our arrangement and presentation of the key themes that were discussed at the conference are inspired by neuroaffective developmental psychology and a neuroaffective view of psychotherapy.

In Chapters One and Two, we introduce our theoretical understanding of the factors that generate transformation processes in psychotherapy with children through the micro-regulation processes that create moments of meeting. In Chapter Two, our focus is on the importance of including the child's primary attachment figures in relation to the organisation of the nervous system and personality development. We also introduce the necessary frame for effective child therapy and the basic principles for neuroaffective developmental psychology, including a look at Paul MacLean's model of the triune brain and the neuroaffective compasses.

In the next four chapters (Chapters Three to Six), we offer brief descriptions of the mental organisations that emerge in the autonomic, limbic, and prefrontal structures. In Chapters One to Three, we also offer a more detailed description of the three neuroaffective compasses.

In Chapter Three, we introduce the autonomic level of organisation and the autonomic compass, along with Peter Levine's somatic experiencing, as this approach is aimed specifically at the autonomic level of organisation. Here we also describe excerpts from two of Levine's demonstration videos. In Chapter Four, we introduce the limbic level of organisation and the limbic compass, along with Jukka Mäkelä's presentation of the Theraplay approach and a transcript of central parts of his demonstration video. In the two following chapters (Chapters Five and Six), we move on to the prefrontal level and to therapies that rely much more on narratives and verbal dialogue. In Chapter Five, we introduce the prefrontal level of organisation and look at regulation in the limbic and prefrontal compass in relation to the Norwegian psychologist Haldor Øvreeide's method of developmentally supportive dialogues with children and his demonstration video. Chapter Six maintains the focus on the prefrontal level, but moves to a higher level of complexity that increases the challenge to the mentalizing capacity. We also discuss the mental development process in the brain's second growth spurt, that is, from the age of two until after adolescence, to provide a basic theoretical understanding for the transformation processes on this mental level. Chapter Six also presents Eia Asen's multi-family mentalization-based approach and reviews the demonstration video that he showed at the conference.

Next, Chapters Seven to Eleven systematically explore the intriguing themes related to the non-specific factors in child psychotherapy that were discussed at the conference. Chapter Seven focuses on the role of the therapist as a good "caravan leader", which means that the therapist should show confidence and leadership to enable the child to trust that a person who is more mature and more highly developed is capable of guiding the child and instilling hope of positive change. Chapter Eight discusses how the symmetrical relationship can unfold in practice, that is, how the therapist can vitalise and "enact" the therapeutic process by means of present moments. The focus of Chapter Nine is on the magical character of the therapeutic process with children, and how this magical process transforms and drives development processes. Chapter Ten looks at the relationship between emotions, words, and mentalization, while Chapter Eleven describes the role of working with the parents in connection with child therapy.

We hope that these chapters will inspire the many professionals who are passionate about assisting parents who have difficulty supporting their children's emotional development, helping them to create good relations to strengthen and mature the child's personality through multiple present moments.

# CHAPTER ONE

# The importance of present moments

"Authenticity comes from the moment, not from the generalisations"

(Jukka Mäkelä)

A s mentioned in the introduction, Daniel Stern, Ed Tronick, Louis Sander, and others formed the Boston Change Study Group in the mid-1990s. They set out to explore the non-specific factors in psychotherapy; in other words: what are the factors in the psychotherapeutic context that are effective but not part of a specific method or among the elements that the psychotherapist emphasises or pays particular attention to in the meeting with the client? As Louis Sander had previously observed, at a very early stage the parent–child dyad synchronises through microscopic moments of meeting and becomes the source of the child's self-regulating processes. Thus, the child in fact develops self-regulation processes by connecting with a more mature and better regulated nervous system. In this chapter, we examine the relevance of so-called present moments for the child's development of a self-regulation capacity and a mature personality. We also examine how we can learn to spot these moments in the psychotherapy process.

## *From regulation to self-organisation*

The nervous system is a complex system, which transforms itself in stops and starts in a process that involves the development of new adaptive forms but also preserves its own continuity. Changes occur in a non-linear fashion, and no one can predict the moment when change is going to occur or the specific form that the development will take. Development represents a new element that emerges as a result of the nervous system's self-organisation and might push it into a new state. The capacity for self-regulation processes is mediated by deep-seated neural structures. The regulation mechanisms in the brain of a newborn child are influenced by the neurochemistry of the nervous system, and the endocrine regulation mechanisms that control brain growth are, in turn, influenced by stimulation from the carer. Feelings and expressions of pleasure and displeasure arise deep inside the subcortical structures, and vocal expressions and emotions, as well as the later emerging cognitive competences that enable speech, depend on regulation in deep-seated subcortical structures in and around the brainstem and inside the limbic system. The emergence of structures in the limbic system transforms self-regulation of arousal into emotions that motivate action. As the nervous system matures, it comes to favour a certain organisation and a certain environmental context, and it seeks previously integrated patterns (Sander, 1977, 1983, 1988).

As Colwyn Trevarthen concludes, the integrative mechanisms for emotions are seated in the subcortical areas that emerge from the brainstem through the cranial nerves and connect with the autonomic nervous system, which regulates arousal, among other functions. Attention focus, including the infant's ability to focus on objects that capture his or her interest, helps provide experiences about the world outside the body and develops along with motor control of body movements. The combination of arousal and attention focus lets the infant attune with another person; this is characterised as the intersubjective capacity. The co-ordination of expressions that carry communicative value is evident from birth, and the internalisation of the intersubjective regulating interactions give rise to a creative self where the child is able to create meaning through pretend play.

At the conference, Peter Levine echoed Colwyn Trevarthen's point that the child's capacity for self-regulation springs from autonomic or central regulation in the brainstem, which also regulates basic functions such as heart rate and breathing and serves as the seat of reflexes and instincts. He described how, when he was studying psychology in the 1960s, the cerebellum was said to be exclusively devoted to the co-ordination of movement; however, today we know that the cerebellum is a crucial structure for the integration of the entire nervous system and for feelings of flow and interpersonal connectedness, and that the area is closely linked to neural structures involved in our perception of sound and touch. The infant's capacity for self-regulation emerges from the neural structures that mediate reflexes, and the maturation of these structures is crucial for personality development. The development of the self-regulation capacity deep inside the basic subcortical structures shapes the organism's fundamental sense of trust and security. This regulation determines, for example, our tendency to approach or avoid something or someone, to freeze in fear, or to bond with another person.

From an early age, the infant responds to others' emotional states; from birth, the child is sensitive to emotions in vocal expressions and touch. The infant is able to express clear emotions and displays a particular curiosity towards human faces. At six months of age, the child is sensitive to the timing of experiences and has the agency to co-ordinate with others' movements. The child responds with greater emotional intensity to rhythms in human body movements, human sounds, and music, and this playful behaviour and body activity act as a highly expressive instrument that is a precursor of the creative imitation that is so characteristic of slightly older children's play and of the imaginative stories with plots and emotions that emerge later. This forms the basis for the conscious and emotional understanding that underpins all cultural intelligence, including language.

From the outset, the carer and the child are interrelated and typically co-ordinate their activities. They engage in an attuned dyadic process in a tremendously flexible manner with room for a high degree of variation that comes to shape the integration and differentiation of the nervous system (Thelen & Smith, 1994). Our sense of "being in the world" is framed by interaction experiences and embedded in neural circuits. Existing neural circuits are modified by current experiences, and, in that sense, what happens now has the power to alter our perception of the past. Ideally, a successful therapeutic process reorganises and integrates the neural circuits that have been shaped by inappropriate regulation strategies in the past (Freeman, 1995; Morgan, 1998).

Louis Sander introduced the term "moments of meeting" in the 1950s, based on the bio-rhythms that begin with the mother–child interaction around the establishment of sleep, waking, and feeding rhythms, and which depend on the carer's and child's engagement in shared activities. He pointed out that the feeling of connectedness, of being on the same wavelength as someone else, springs from the influence that the carer and the infant have on one another during the first six months after the child's birth, which emerges in mutually synchronised regulation where the carer's and the infant's respective nervous systems engage in a reciprocal field of resonance. The synchronisation of the carer's and the infant's nervous systems takes place through moments of meeting, which play a crucial role for the organisation of the brain and for the central nervous system's regulatory processes.

Sander also pointed out that moments of meeting increase the nervous system's capacity for intensifying and co-regulating with another person's activities. These moments only arise when the infant's and the carer's nervous systems have been able to engage in a process of mutual adjustment and self-regulation that Daniel Stern calls "moving along". In the moments of meeting, the infant's and the carer's states of mind are connected, resulting in a mutual recognition where they share a sense of the other's experience. For example, when a mother and an infant engage in a well-regulated interaction, a particular smile from the child that she finds surprising or amusing may make her look at the child with a big smile that makes them both laugh. When a moment of meeting occurs, the attunement is at full intensity, and there is an overwhelming feeling of intimacy and authenticity. These moments are crucial for nourishing the nervous system and stimulating development (Sander, 1992; Stern, 1977, 1998a, 2004).

The transfer of emotional information is intensified through these present moments, or moments of meeting, and the heightened energy leads to a sense of vitality that develops the nervous system's emergent capacity for self-regulation and attention control. If, for example, a carer and an infant are playing and an exchange of laughter escalates and pushes both the carer and the infant to a higher level of arousal, this will increase the infant's capacity for tolerating higher levels of mutually generated positive arousal in future interactions.

Tiny changes that occur at the right time stimulate the nervous system to reorganise and develop (Sander, 1988; Schore, 2003a,b; Sroufe, 1996; Stern, 1990, 1998a).

The desire to be in an intersubjective field with another person is an important condition for the formation of relations and is one of the factors driving the psychotherapeutic process. The intersubjective field can only emerge in the moment, and when it does, it gives rise to emotional moments where personal resources are built and where the person shows a higher degree of flexibility and stronger mental health. Mental states are reflected in the behaviour of the two participants, and their meeting in this shared moment expands both parties' experience. Virtually all humans possess this potential for emotional bonding. As Stern (2004) points out, we develop our emotional capacity by living in the present in the framework of implicitly learnt dyadic interactions.

Tronick has pointed out that the infant is a subsystem within a larger dyadic system that is regulated by the other subsystem, the carer's, which shapes the infant's limited regulatory capacity. This insight can be applied to the therapeutic process. For example, the therapist supports a regulation of the child's affect in a mutual dyadic mental state regulation, where the child and the therapist together form new and more complex exchanges that shape the child's self-confidence as well as the child's trust in the therapist. Even though change is threatening, because it is unpredictable, it also implies hope. The motivation to establish an emotional attachment is innate and intrinsic. When two individuals fail to attune emotionally, there is no development.

## Establishing regulatory attachment experiences through a process of improvisation

Trevarthen (1993a,b) explains that social knowledge is produced through interaction, and even infants possess a rudimentary version of this capacity. The motivation to establish emotional attachment is an innate, intrinsic capacity. In childhood, intersubjective processes are an inseparable part of self-organisation processes, and the human brain has adapted to engage in intersubjective development and cultural learning. Neural structures for self-preservation and self-co-ordination regulate themselves through the structures that ensure mutual co-ordination between self and others. In any dyad, whether it is the carer–child relationship or the therapist–child relationship, the nervous system is a self-organising system that creates its own states of brain organisation, and by co-operating with another self-organising system the child can develop highly complex states.

Sander (1977) describes that when two persons' directionalities come together, a transformation process ensues that enables new development. As described by Winnicott in his clinical observations, this occurs when both parties reach a moment of joint attention where the child becomes aware that another person is aware of what the child is aware of within him/herself. Winnicott has called this "the sacred moment", a moment of meeting that involves a new degree of coherence in the child's experience of his or her attention to inner states as well as the external world. In this process, the child has the experience of both "being with" and "being different from" another person. Throughout life, this synchronisation occurs in a matter of microseconds, generating positive affect and engagement and moving the child and the carer towards shared experiences. The infant's capacity for self-organising preferred states and goals produces a sense of being different from that promotes the development of a separate identity. Adaptation establishes self-regulation based on the recognition of inner experiences—of subjectivity and intersubjectivity (Hart, 2011).

The bond between two nervous systems involves a dyadic form of resonance, where energy and information can flow freely, which is the source of present moments, or moments of meeting. These moments occur suddenly and spontaneously; they are easy to see, difficult to describe verbally, and they are probably the moments when the child truly feels met, and where a transformation can take place that moves the child from one level of development to the next. The present moments are co-created by the two parties in the relationship and require an emotional openness from them both. For these meetings to occur, there has to be a mutual recognition of the other's feelings, and each party has to understand and confirm what unfolds between them. The present moment provides openness and a sense of belonging that activates the brain's subcortical areas, which are related to affects about emotions (Sander, 1992).

Present moments are steps in a process of moving along, they are typically brief and consist of the time that is needed for both individuals to develop a sense of what is happening between them, right now. The repeated, musically interlocking activities of the parent–child interaction allow them both gradually to build a repertoire of present moments, forming a familiar register of how the lived moments in life with a specific other can be expected to unfold in the process of moving along (Stern, 1998a). Present moments that are linked together create a process of moving along in a shared improvisation with a sense of approaching a goal. Each step in this process of moving along is a present moment where a unit of subjective time plays out a motif aimed at micro-regulating the content and objectives of psychotherapy and adjusting the intersubjectivity. The therapeutic change process often consists of numerous undramatic moments of meeting with perhaps a few dramatic ones interwoven.

Often, small changes lead to major changes (Morgan, 1998). The small changes are created through the dramatic present moments and carry affective importance for the therapeutic process. In these moments, the therapist and the child are drawn more actively into the moment, and something important emerges that helps shape the future. When this moment is seized, that is, when both the therapist and the child display authentic, personal responses, it can be assumed that they both share the same experience and have a mutual experience of sharing the same mental landscape. In the context of the carer–child interaction, Stern (1998a,b) describes how a funny expression or a surprising incident can trigger a synchronisation where both participants burst out laughing simultaneously. The interaction leaps to a higher level of activation, and the child experiences an unprecedented fullness of joy that goes beyond any previously shared experience. This altered state enables new mental conceptions and actions and the reorganisation of previous events.

## The importance of synchronisation and micro-regulation processes

Sander describes that we come into the world with two innate biological motivations that shape the fit between the child and carer. One is the need to synchronise and self-regulate the endogenous biological mechanisms that maintain vital functions, the other is the capacity for interpersonal synchronicity through microsecond-long attunements with another. These innate mechanisms are present from the beginning of life and ensure important conditions for the internal self-regulation capacities that develop through attachment experiences. This synchronisation process is experienced as positive affect and develops an inner motivation system that forms the basis for "healthy" relationships, including the experience of giving and receiving love. This experience also enables us to synchronise with others later in life and to recognise the experience of attachment. The shared intense focus of attention that is created in moments of meeting enables the essential attunement processes that occur in microseconds. The base of experiences that develops as a result of the attunement processes organises the formation of consciousness. Relationships are based on connectedness, and we embark on life being connected, being part of someone else—in other words, we begin our lives in a relationship.

The dyadic regulation of states between two individuals is based on micro-exchanges of information through perceptual systems and affective properties as they unfold and are responded to by the carer and the child over time. Regulation includes intensification, down-regulation, processing, repairs, and establishment as well as a return to a pre-set equilibrium. The carer's ability to understand the infant's state and to synchronise with this state is one of the factors that determine the nature and degree of coherence with the infant's experiences. The change in the therapeutic relationship also occurs through microscopic moments of meeting, which leave their marks in microscopic changes to the neural circuits.

Rigid and inflexible patterns can be difficult to change, and certain neural patterns that emerge as a result of traumatic events may be immune to what happens in the moment. Previous events have a radical impact on the present, and altering existing neural circuits can prove a long and arduous process, although, as a universal principle, the present is constantly rewriting the past. Sometimes, neurophysiological changes can be so irreversibly ingrained early in life through critical periods and severe traumas and conflicts that they prove very resistant to change (Gunnar & Vazquez, 2001).

Physiobiological and psychobiological regulation begins immediately after birth. The carer provides psychological coherence in a regulation process that unfolds from one second to the next. In early regulation, vocalisation soon takes on a key role, and the rhythm and tonality of the voice has a direct influence on psychobiological moti-vation. In the therapeutic process, the therapist similarly provides a caring context that facilitates growth and development. By establish-ing an alliance and empathic attunement with the child, the therapist seeks to activate attachment processes, modulate anxiety and stress levels, and create an optimal biochemical environment that promotes neural plasticity. When internal or external factors hinder the child's ability to approach challenging, stressful situations, the neural system tends to remain underdeveloped and unintegrated.

Within the framework of the psychotherapeutic relationship, the therapist attempts to modify the micro-anatomy of the child's brain. Once an autonomic or limbic connection has been established as a neural pattern, it can only be modified by an autonomic or a limbic connection. To achieve the integration and reintegration of neural circuits, the nervous system needs to connect with another nervous system and enter into a field of resonance with it. Successful attune-ment lets the nervous system develop flexibility and integrate neural patterns that are dispersed throughout the hierarchic organisation of the brain. Dyadic communication enables resonance and coherence in the nervous system. Development and integration emerge in a balance between care and optimal stress. Moderate arousal or optimal stress levels are necessary to integrate and consolidate neural circuits, provided the stress level does not exceed the capacity of the nervous system. An activation of the nervous system beyond this level triggers a powerful sympathetic activation that inhibits cortical processing and disturbs the integrative functions. Conversely, moderate sympathetic arousal intensifies the capacity of the neural network to process and integrate information. The therapeutic process combines emotionally calm and agitated moments, reflecting the underlying neural rhythm for growth and change. Optimal levels of arousal and stress result in an increased release of neurotransmitters and neural growth hor-mones, which enhances learning and cortical reorganisation, and a successful therapeutic process leads to the development of neural circuits (Cozolino, 2002).

As Peter Levine explained at the conference, interventions are often very simple and based on micro-changes. There is often a high degree of repetitiveness in what the therapist says and does and in the use of certain words with profound impact and meaning. In Levine's opinion, this sort of repetition is one of the highly effective non-specific factors in therapy. Repetitions unfold a new resource, a new-found experience that subsequent experiences build on. Repetitions establish a rhythm that keeps the flow going. Jukka Mäkelä referred to this as the small elements of the present moment that create the dyadic expansion of consciousness: "Knowing that there is something bigger that we are approaching when we are together, where things happen that we don't quite understand." Although we can never predict the magic of what happens, it is driven by "the shared under-standing that I am here, you are here, and there is something going on between us, and in that 'something' things happen which I am not in control of, and you don't have to be in control of, but we can trust that life builds integration. And this is, I think, what all therapy is about."

## The role of attunement, misattunement, and the repair of misattunements

Affective attunement and affirmation are part of being seen and appreciated, and, undoubtedly, this interactive process drives person-ality development. In attuned contacts, information is transmitted about the other's inner world, and when two people allow a field of resonance to emerge, they can develop a sense of what it is like inside the other's emotional world. To feel that one is seen by another person or to feel emotionally acknowledged is the first step in an emotional development process and in the transformation of personal experi-ences (Hart, 2010; Lewis, Amini, & Lannon, 2001; Schibbye, 2005).

Resonance plays a crucial role in the organisation of the brain and in the regulatory processes of the central nervous system. Resonance means that the activation of something triggers resonant effects that, in turn, intensify the activity. Sander (1977) has argued that infants begin life with an endogenous rhythmic activity that needs to be co-ordinated with a partner, and that the nervous system contains a biological motivating drive to organise information, discover regu-larity, and act on the basis of expectations. This inner process is organised by the nervous system in mutual regulation with another nervous system, and these shared experiences gradually form the basis for intimacy, attachment, mutual attunement, self-regulation, and self-reflection. In this mutual transfer, one connects the observed behaviour of a partner, for example, a facial expression, with one's own inner mental state and perception (Beebe & Lachmann, 2002). The human nervous system seeks to discover the experiences of others by creating fields of resonance with them. Individuals with a well-integrated nervous system engage in fields of resonance with each other's intentions, feelings, and thoughts, which, in turn, are constantly modified or created in dialogues with others' felt intentions. The nervous system is designed to allow us to experience another person's nervous system from within by creating a field of resonance with their nervous system and, thus, share their experiences. The human nervous system is emotionally affected by someone else's behaviour, which is the basis of empathy (Hart, 2010; Stern, 2004).

In the therapeutic process, the therapist has to be able to enter into vitalising positive attunement with the child. The core of empathy is the capacity for matching the other's affect and providing a resonant response. Positive attunement builds trust and drives the establishment of attachment bonds. Through resonance and synchronicity, the therapist forms attachment bonds with the child and, thus, supports the child's implicit (unconscious) recognition of previous relationship strategies that have constituted an obstacle to psychological development. When the therapist is empathically attuned with the child's inner state, the contact is intensified and vitalised (Hammer, 1990; Hart, 2010; Schore, 2003b; Stern, 1984; Trevarthen, 1979).

Moving along in therapy is a spontaneous and unpredictable process, and it might be difficult for an outside observer to discern any particular direction. This unpredictable process is only potentially creative, however, when it unfolds within a well-established framework, which is achieved when the therapist uses a method that he or she feels comfortable with. Stern (2004) points out the need to work within a specific technique and theoretical guidelines for the events that unfold to be meaningful. Bowlby described that the best therapist is someone who is naturally intuitive, that is, a therapist who is able to use his or her subjective implicit experience, and who is guided by the appropriate theory (Bowlby, 1991; Schore, 2003b).

Connecting in an intersubjective space necessitates a series of spontaneous exchanges as well as multiple misunderstandings and misattunements. Even the very best interactions include many misattunements, but the vast majority are quickly repaired by both parties. These misattunements are valuable because they develop our capacity for tolerating frustration and for repairing and reattuning misattunements; these little mishaps are, therefore, essential for getting to know each other. Early on, Tronick realised the importance of re-establishing attunement after a misattunement in a mutually regulating repair process. These shifts from an attuned to a mis-attuned state and from a misattuned to an attuned state occur every three to five seconds.

An infant who fails to apply his or her coping strategies and who is repeatedly unable to repair misattunements begins to feel help-less. The infant will gradually give up trying to repair misattunements and instead increasingly base his or her coping strategies on self-regulation in an attempt to control the negative experiences caused by a failure to establish contact. The infant internalises a pattern of coping strategies that limit his or her engagement with the social envi-ronment and develops a negative self-perception as well as a negative perception of the environment. Ironically, when the child applies this coping strategy in potentially normal interactions, these interactions, too, become distorted. This leads to a self-perpetuating cycle, which might gradually become a personality pattern that leads to significant psychological difficulties. Self-regulation and interactive regulation are two aspects of the regulation process.

In the 1970s, Tronick introduced his "still face" experiment, and, over the years, he has carried out this experiment with hundreds of infants aged from around three months to one year. In the video recordings, he saw the unfolding of the child's many coping strategies for handling the mother's failure to respond to the child's signals. Some children were very persistent in their attempts to coax a res-ponse from the mother with smiles and positive vocalisations. Others used negative affect, and some a combination of both. Some children looked at their mother, but soon turned their attention to an object without turning back to the mother. Some displayed stress signals in the form of rapid, shallow breathing, but were unable either to draw out the mother or turn towards an object. Instead, they attempted to self-soothe by staring into thin air. Interactive stress can be caused by a wide variety of factors, from a bad timing of emotional signals, a misinterpretation of signals, or different goals to over- or under-stimulation. Interactive stress occurs because mother and infant are unable to maintain mutual regulation throughout an interaction period. The infant's first reactions to the "still face" experiment occur within the first two seconds. Even after the mother has resumed normal interaction, the infant remains affected by the experience for some time. There is less eye contact, and the child's mood remains dampened for several minutes. Even three-month-old infants are influenced not only by the mother's immediate response or lack of response, but also by the overarching event that causes a more persistent mood.

As described in the introduction to Tronick's chapter in *Neuro-affektiv psykoterapi med børn* (Hart, 2011), normal mother–child interactions are constantly moving from one misattunement to the next, alternating with successful repairs. The child's experiences of repairing normal misattuned states have a profound impact on the child's coping strategies when he or she is subjected to the more extreme stress of encountering the mother's expressionless face. In the "still face" experiment, the infants who were used to engaging in successful mutual regulations with their mothers were also better at displaying positive signals, their signals were less negative, and they were not as disorganised as the children who were less used to experiencing repairs of misattunement processes.

When mothers were asked to tone down their facial expressions, speak in a monotonous tone of voice, move slowly, and sit some distance away from the infant, the infants were more affected than they were by the "still face" experiment, probably because the mothers' behaviour does have a degree of attunement with the child's but is poorly matched and produces multiple misattunements. The children of more intrusive mothers, for example, mothers with many angry outbursts directed at the child, tended to avert their gaze more. In contrast, mothers who tended to face away from their infants, had children who were more maladjusted and who protested more. Behaviours such as averting one's gaze and sucking on a thumb can calm down a distressed infant and help control the child's negative emotions. That lets the child shift his or her attention away from the disturbing incident, which slows down the heart rate.

Normal infants in normal interactions with adults experience a high rate of misattunements in the interaction, but they have the coping strategies to handle them and, thus, preserve their self-regulation capacity. This capacity stabilises around the age of six months. The experience of being able to repair interactive misattunements and negative emotions has developmental advantages that produce positive emotions. It enables the child to maintain his or her engagement with the environment, even in stressful situations, and to develop clearer boundaries between self and other. As early as at the age of six months, the infant is able to display an affective coping style and a representation of self and other.

Tronick observed a link, albeit an incomplete one, between the mutual regulation of infant–carer interactions and therapist–client/ child interactions. He noted that the therapy process includes the same number of attunement and misattunement processes as the infant–carer interaction, and that the therapeutic relationship also consists of two individuals engaged in an active effort to create coherent meaning. In the Boston Change Study Group, Tronick argued the need to focus more on the repair of misattunements than on synchronisation as the transformative process in psychotherapy and development. Many changes occur in the moments of meeting when a misattunement becomes an attunement process. When new information is selectively incorporated, it produces a feeling of expansion and joy. An increased degree of complexity causes the child to feel more connected to the therapist, and the relationship becomes deeper. In turn, the child feels a deeper sense of self, which is accompanied by a feeling of solidarity, stability, and self-continuity. This expansion of consciousness is a powerful experience.

Attunement, selective attunement, and misattunement are ways of conveying attitudes, fantasies, and plans. Attunement can be used for both good and bad purposes, but in either case it opens intersubjective doors between people and provides a partial union with another human being. It has the capacity to enrich our mental life, but also to restrict it by bending an aspect of an inner experience in a particular direction or excluding it. Selective attunement contributes to changing the child's subjective experience by emphasising certain aspects of the experience and toning down others. Stern calls misattunements "missteps in the dance" and deems them highly valuable because negotiation and repairs within the interaction are among the most important ways of conveying the rules for being with another person. The correction of missteps develops into the child's coping strategies. The process of missteps and repairs is one of the most essential learning experiences for the child in interacting with an imperfect world. Missteps are helpful because they require the child to perform a coping or adjustment manoeuvre in order to correct, alter, or avoid a troubling situation. In order to develop, the infant needs constant practice in adapting his or her behaviour to ever-changing conditions. The carer contributes to this process by ensuring the child's ability to expand his or her stimulus tolerance.

As mentioned above, selective attunements help to shape the child's subjective experience by emphasising certain aspects of the experience over others. Some of these selective attunements are called social referencing. That occurs when children experience insecure situations, for example, when the child is involved in an exercise that he or she is uncertain about. In these ambiguous situations, the child will look at the therapist, scanning his or her face for affective content in order to determine what would be an appropriate feeling and secure a second opinion to resolve the ambiguity. Social referencing, to some extent, allows the carer or the therapist to decide and influence the child's actual experience. A certain degree of attunement is necessary to enable successful social referencing. Affective attunement lets child know whether his or her experiences are shared by the carer and, thus, are part of a shared world.

### Anchoring therapy in the present moment and using RIGS to activate the episodic memory

In the carer–child interaction, many activities are repeated in an improvisation process that comes to represent schemas for ways of being with others. Stern (1998b) points out that children require special care which adults have to offer (Stern, 1998b). Cognition research has found that representations, memories, and motor patterns do not exist in a fixed, final, and absolute form that is only waiting to be triggered or activated; instead, they are composed or constructed anew every time they are brought into the working memory, based on the requirements of the given context. Stern describes that whatever happens in the present moment will activate all the networks of schemas at all the hierarchical levels that have any mental or physical connection to the current ongoing activity.

Virtually all types of interaction behaviour are governed by an activated schema that is involved in selecting and shaping the actual interactive behaviour that is displayed. On the other hand, interactive behaviour also activates schemas for being-with, and, once a schema has been activated, its actual manifestation depends on the given context. A shared experience is a moment that is constructed by the participants' mental system as it unfolds in the moment. We experience ourselves as being in the moment and create a draft of what is happening, which is then represented in schemas for being-with. In that sense, representations are based on subjectively perceived interaction experiences.

As Stern describes it, episodes are stored in memory as indivisible units. Ordinarily, an episode appears a distinctive whole, an episodic memory. If several similar episodes occur, the child forms a representation of a generalised episode. This generalised memory is an individualised and personal expectation of how things are likely to change from one moment to the next. Generalised episodes serve as basic building blocks, both in cognitive development and in our autobiographic memory. Interaction experiences revolve around actions, sensory impressions, and emotions that are represented in a preverbal form, and, in Stern's terminology, they constitute "representations of interactions that have been generalised" (RIGs). RIGs are flexible structures that represent averages of multiple actual experiences. This means that they are not specific memories, but abstractions based on many specific memories, which, although they differ slightly, produce a generalised memory structure. According to Stern, most specific memories are summarised and lost in this generalisation process. Many memories are not limited to one event in the past but, instead, represent the accumulated history of a particular type of interaction. The prototypical memories have a guiding function, as the past produces expectations of the present and the future.

The experience of being with a self-regulating other gradually forms RIGs. As different RIGs are activated, the infant relives different ways of being with the regulating other. Each memory is unique because it is triggered by a specific context, which will never repeat itself in exactly the same way. For each of the different memory contexts that are selected in the moment, a different set of fragments will be selected, or the same set will be put together in a different way. With inspiration from a professor of neurophysiology, Walter Freeman, Stern describes that as each new present moment is formed, the neural representation of the past is altered and the possible memories of the past are revised. The original memory tracks have been altered and no longer exist in their original form. The past is constantly revised and, in a sense, we could say that the present is gradually altering the past. To illustrate, Stern mentions an example from Freeman, who showed that when rabbits are exposed to a new smell, a neural activation pattern is established. When the rabbit is later exposed to another new smell, a new neural activation pattern is established for this new smell. The establishment of the second activation pattern alters the neural activation pattern associated with the first smell. Later, when the rabbit is exposed to a third smell, both of the two previous patterns are altered. In that sense, the past is always being permanently revised, both as a neural pattern and as an experience of recall. However, Stern also mentions that severely traumatising experiences could produce inflexible patterns that appear resistant to change from new present experiences.

A specific singular episode will always result in altering the RIG, which is updated on an ongoing basis. All the interactions we have taken part in are internalised in the form of RIGs; Stern calls these internalised relations evoked companions. An evoked companion is an activated memory from one or more RIGs that are evoked by a recall sign of something that occurs right now in the meeting with another person. The evoked companion is part of the episodic memory and typically concerns the emotional side of the contact. Evoked companions never go away, and they are active both in concrete interactions and in the other's absence in the form of an active memory. Evoked companions can be activated by bodily sensations or emotions, and, over time, they may activate self-regulating strategies that might facilitate psychological development.

Links among related RIGs form networks of internalised representations, which are integrated into increasingly comprehensive interpersonal experiences of being with the other person—that is to say, a wide variety of evoked companions. Once an internal representation has become sufficiently comprehensive, it has become a relationship that exists in consciousness, and consciousness brings a story of the relationship with it into every new interactive experience and influences the course of every new interaction. When a new interactive event has been internalised, the experienced story can alter the internal representation. This produces a dynamic interaction between past and present, between established internal representations and present exchanges, between the relationship and the ongoing interaction. The relational process never ends, even in adulthood.

The child's relationships and internal representations are constantly expanded, altered, and transformed through RIGs, a process that is utilised in psychotherapy. Attunement, selective attunements, and misattuned processes lead to the formation of RIGs, which form evoked companions and self-regulating "others" in the child's mind. Limbic circuits develop through stimulation, and the child is able to develop his or her full limbic potential only when he or she enters into an affectively attuned contact. The child responds emotionally to others as if they represent important persons from the past, and the impact of previous events might distort new attunements. In the psychotherapeutic process, the therapist gradually seeks to alter these RIGs by means of more appropriate attunement processes (Hart & Schwartz, 2008).

An important non-specific factor in psychotherapy concerns how we, as human beings, generally include others in our emotional reality. We do this through emotional attunement, which triggers implicit memories and emotional states in both ourselves and others. When we engage in interactions, we are attracted to each other's emotional world, we attune emotionally with each other, and, thus, influence each other. Our understanding of others is reflected back and might influence the other's self-concept and alter neural circuits. Emotional resonance lets us understand both our own and others' inner world. In a sense, a mutual regulation of mental states occurs between the therapist and the child. This regulation takes place in a relationship characterised by an asymmetric distribution of responsibility, where the therapist supports the child's restructuring and, thus, the modification of the child's mental organisation in a sort of mutual expansion of consciousness. Thus, it is not symbolisation or interpretation that alters the mind, although they can help if they are timed properly; it is the synchronisation that occurs in the procedural, implicit part of the brain that produces the actual transformation processes. These are the processes that regulate the child's mental state awareness of how to enter into other relationships, that is, how to regulate in relation to others. The capacity for establishing mutual states with others and the quality of these exchanges basically depend on the child's previous capacity for creating these states with others, originally with the primary carers. This also means that it is not verbal narratives, such as the memory of something one's mother did, that change one's way of relating to others; instead, it is the mutual regulation that we are accustomed to and expect will affect our present emotional and relational interactions. It is the process of moving along and the present moments that enable the development of a more complex and coherent way of being with significant others.

## The development of a capacity for affect regulation and personality maturation through synchronised present moments

Stern describes that co-regulation really requires that the carer falls in love with the child, and the child falls in love with the carer. This state is rarely in place from the outset, but emerges gradually through a process of improvisation. A carer should trust her own innate maternal behaviour, and, in order to maintain the child's interest and arousal, she needs to improvise and vary her actions. It is this process that needs to be moved into the therapy room. Psychotherapy, which is based on emotional resonance, pursues this process through improvised interactions. Most of the time, the interaction unfolds in a basic back-and-forth exchange, and suddenly there is an intense shift: the present moment. This interaction between two persons requires an attentive and authentic presence where the implicit knowledge between the therapist and the child is allowed to fuse. Both the therapist and the child should be able to move freely in the process, and there should be time for fun if any transformation is to take place (Stern, 2001).

The past influences the experiences that are formed in the present. In therapy, the goal is to alter the internal representations of the past to enable the person to select different elements that might influence the future. We live in the present, and the experiences we acquired in the past unfold in the present. The present moment is thus the place where past and present come together. The part of the past that influences the present can be reorganised in the intersubjective meeting, which consists of a series of present moments (Stern, 2004). As mentioned earlier, it is in the present moments that the child becomes aware that another person is aware of what the child is aware of inside him/herself (Sander, 1995). Hence, the present moments are healing and identity forming and capable of altering the brain's organisation. They contribute to neural coherence and to the development of self-regulating strategies. The mutual affirmation of one another's gaze makes each partner present in his or her own right. This is the core of identity development, and if the child is not met in this form of affirmation, there is no room for his or her identity to unfold.

In therapy, present moments repeat variations on the familiar interactions in a relationship, which shape the unique interaction in a therapeutic dyad. In normal communication, including the communication that takes place in the therapy room, one or both parties will often fail to be present in the moment because their focus shifts to the past or the future, or other aspects of the present. When that happens, the present moments do not occur. To move the development forward, the therapist has to dare to meet the moment with an authentic response that is spontaneous and carries his or her personal signature. In a present moment, the therapy moves into a new improvisation process, but in an expanded mutual field that allows new possibilities. The affective state signals whether the parties have arrived at a place where the therapeutic process is able to move forward (Stern, 1998b, 2001; Stern et al., 1998). Drawing on his or her intuition, the therapist senses when a change occurs that has the potential to develop into a present moment or a moment of meeting. The relationship does the work and, thus, therapy hinges on establishing a safe environment where we have room to unfold our internal representations. The emotional attunement allows co-regulation, and the neural circuit that is activated in the present moment determines which parts of the past are activated and how pre-existing elements are combined to match the present situation.

The present moment alters the *functional* past, not the *historical* past. Recognition memories are established in relation to experiences in the moment. They involve, for example, the recognition of a smell, a sound, a melody, a word, etc., which is integrated into the given moment. Every moment of recognition is a slightly different experience, as different fragments are selected in relation to what is happening in the moment (Stern, 2004). Internal representations come together, break up, and come together again in relation to the moment of the event (Beebe & Lachmann, 2002). As Peter Levine mentioned at the conference, the normal developmental process contains general or non-specific elements, and sticking to those normal developmental principles or factors in the communication with the child and the parents can produce very specific outcomes. The outcomes are specific to *this* child under *these* circumstances in *this* situation in the life condition that the child is currently stuck in. Haldor Øvreeide mentioned the importance of the therapist following the child, rather than pushing for his or her own ideas. Jukka Mäkelä added that, since it is the non-specific factors that create the specific outcomes, a psychotherapist needs to know what the intended goal is and what is being created in the developmental process. There has to be a structure, for example, in the form of a particular game or activity, such as popping soap bubbles, a kind of substance or structure that leads to something and which makes the child feel safe enough to follow along and offer up his or her own initiatives. Simply offering "open love" or stress release will fail to bring out the normal developmental principles. In an unstructured offer, no one is leading the process, and that can be extremely frightening for a child. As Peter Levine pointed out, personality development is much more about the personal meeting than it is about trauma or symptom release.

## Summary

In this chapter, we have discussed how the co-ordination of expressions that have communicative value is evident from birth, and how the internalisation of intersubjective regulatory interactions enable the development of a creative self. At the age of six months, the infant is sensitive to the timing of experiences, and, through his or her own agency, the child is able to co-ordinate with others' movements and responds more emotionally to rhythms in human body movements, human sounds, and music. Even within the first six months of life, the infant develops a sense of being connected with, or on the same wavelength as, the carer through the mutual influence that carer and child have on one another, and they establish a mutual field of resonance through temporally synchronised co-regulation.

The self-regulation capacity develops in a process of attunement, misattunement, and repair of misattunement framed by a string of present moments that generate synchronicity in mutual interactions that stimulate neural structures. Throughout life, this synchronisation continues to unfold in micro-seconds, creating positive affect and engagement that move the child and the carer towards being together. To feel seen by someone else and being emotionally recognised are the first steps in an emotional developmental process. The child's desire to be in an intersubjective field with another person is important for building the relationship and also helps to drive the psychotherapy process.

The child's relationships and internal representations are constantly expanded, altered, and transformed through so-called RIGs. RIGs create new episodic memories and may gradually alter previous interaction experiences through the present moments; they are formed through synchronised processes, which help to shape self-regulating "others" in the child's awareness. The psychotherapy process aims to alter these RIGs gradually through more adaptive attunement processes.

# CHAPTER TWO

# Neuroaffective developmental psychology: a "map" for understanding child psychotherapy

"If a method fails to create now-moments, it's not the right method, even if the therapist might think it is. Therapy should bring vitality to the autonomic and the limbic system before the words can connect to mentalisation"

(Hart & Bentzen)

To understand the non-specific factors in child psychotherapy, we think it is necessary to understand the key supportive context that surrounds the child's personality development, that is, the importance of family and primary carers, and how the child's normal development unfolds in this context through macro- and micro-regulatory processes. In this chapter, we look at the important role of the primary carers and also offer a brief description of the natural development of mental organisations, since the transformations that occur in therapy have to relate to this context. With inspiration from MacLean's triune model of the brain (1990), we describe these maturation processes in the framework of neuroaffective developmental psychology, which we consider particularly crucial, as the child's emotional neural structures mature within the framework of the child's developmental capacity or, in other words, within the child's zone of proximal development.

## The child as part of a larger relational context

As early as the 1960s, Bowlby pointed out that all the things that carers routinely do for their children are taken so much for granted that we fail to see their importance. Being the carer of a child, he said, is not something that can be put into a formalised schedule; it is a living human relationship that transforms both parties' personality. He explained that although the attachment behaviour is especially evident in early childhood, it remains a key characteristic of human life from cradle to grave. In our understanding, this also applies to the non-specific factors in child psychotherapy. Bowlby described how the child constructs internal images of him/herself and others in everyday interactions; he called these constructs internal working models. As the child forms internal representations of attachment experiences and other life experiences, he or she forms an internal secure, or insecure, base that helps to organise the child's behaviour, including behaviours in social relations later in life. Shortcomings in either party's capacity for transmitting or receiving, or flaws in their mutual synchronisation, can disrupt the development process. In addition, traumas, even if they are not necessarily attachment related, such as drowning accidents, etc., can lead to psychological imbalances and disrupt the child's development process. It is exactly this type of psychological imbalance that the psychotherapy process with children aims to resolve.

Winnicott's well-known claim that "there is no such thing as an infant"—meaning that an infant can never exist outside of a relationship—is a key point in relation to child therapy. Winnicott first made this comment at a meeting in the British Psychoanalytical Society around 1940 and later revisited it in a footnote to a 1960 article in which he also wrote that "the infant and the maternal care belong to each other and cannot be disentangled" (Winnicott, 1960, p. 587).

In child psychotherapy, the therapist should always understand the child in relation to his or her closest carers, both in relation to the child's intersubjective and relational competences and in the relationship with the carer. Child or family therapy must, therefore, never lose sight of the child's closest carers.

As is highlighted in the systemic approach (Sameroff, 1989; Sander, 1977, 1983), children's psychological difficulties rarely reside in the child alone but are, instead, embedded in the relationship between a unique child and an environment that is incapable of supporting the experiences that are necessary for the child to self-regulate and to develop more advanced levels of mental organisation. As Sameroff (1989) points out, higher social mammals cannot be understood independently of the relationship of which they are a part. Apart from the carer's significant impact on the child's personality development, it is also important how the other family members relate to each other. Once the child enters nursery or school, another important factor is how the child is seen by teachers, peers, and others. Others' perceptions of the child and of the child's parents and larger family have a huge impact on the child's self-concept and coping strategies. It is in the light of this context that we should understand the child's difficulties in the psychotherapeutic relationship. This points to two essential aspects of child psychotherapy: one is to address the child's psychological imbalances, whether the predisposing factors are conditioned by unattuned relational experiences or by other types of traumatic experiences; the other is to integrate the primary carers.

Salvador Minuchin, who was involved in developing structural family therapy, emphasised how important it is for the health of the family to have a clear generational hierarchy between children and parents. Destructive alliances across the generations lead to dysfunction. The systemic and structural view of the child as the symptom-bearer of family issues is an important concept that highlights the importance of the way in which psychopathology reflects interpersonal or family dynamic relationships. The child needs the adults' recognition and guidance to develop adaptive relational strategies and social skills. The interaction between a child and an adult, whether a parent or a therapist, should be based on an asymmetric distribution of responsibility. When the parents fail to support the child's developmental capacity, it becomes an important therapeutic goal to make sure that the child is seen, with his or her resources and challenges, also by the parents, and to help the parents modify their interactions with the child accordingly.

In our view, this is what happens through the present moments and micro-regulatory interaction processes in psychotherapy described in the previous chapter. As Asen (2005) and others have pointed out, there are many levels in the child's life that need to be integrated to alter the child's psyche and behaviour, including the child's level of functioning, the way the parents relate to the child, the family constellation, the social context the family lives, and the support that the professional system provides for the family.

All children, even children who have been abused, are loyal to their parents and remain attached to them. The child may feel sad, feel unfairly treated, and be stuck in destructive mood swings that rob the child of the opportunity to receive the love he or she yearns for, but the child is still attached to the parents, even if the attachment pattern might be insecure. Even if the child might deny the attachment, he or she often longs to express his or her love and to be loved back. At first, the child's life is organised in the relationship with the carer, but, over time, the child becomes an increasingly active participant and eventually develops behaviours that maintain the pattern. It is these fixated patterns that the psychotherapy process attempts to alter.

## Personality maturation

As described in *Neuroaffektiv psykoterapi med børn* (Hart, 2011), the potential that is present in the nervous system from birth has a crucial impact on individual development. The innate biological capacity enables the child to engage in social interactions and emotional communication because, as human beings, we have a biological predisposition to establish attachment bonds. We are born with a highly plastic nervous system that enables us to interact with the environment we are born into, and our individual personalities develop in a social or attachment-based context.

Although the human brain is self-organising, this organisation process depends on two brain systems, as the child's immature nervous system has a limited capacity for self-organisation, in part due to relatively slow information processing speed, limited motor control, and a limited capacity in the sensory and associative areas of the brain. The relationship promotes the development of a unique pattern of neural circuits. As a result of this process, each human brain is completely unique and shaped by both neurogenesis and environment. The child's responses to stimuli activate specific neurons that form circuits and neural patterns. When this pattern is activated at a later point, it enters into a constant transformation process that alters and reinforces the original pattern. Once a neural circuit has been established, it is easily reactivated by implicit (unconscious) memory tracks. In a neuroaffective sense, the carers' regulation of the child has a direct influence on the child's biochemical growth processes. This forms the basis for the development of new structures, which gradually leads to increasingly well-developed mental organisations. At birth, some neural circuits are fully functional, most are developing, and a few remain undifferentiated. The levels of mental organisation do not change in a linear progression throughout childhood; instead, there are huge leaps and qualitative shifts at certain times (Beebe & Lachmann, 2002; Perry, 2002; Schore, 1994).

Attachment relationships are formative because they promote the development of the brain's self-regulating mechanisms, and if the individual interacts with others to strengthen his or her self-regulation capacity, the self-organising potential will be unfolded. Hierarchical integration co-ordinates each level of mental organisation with previous levels, and reorganisation occurs with the progression of development (Cicchetti & Tucker, 1994; Fonagy, 1998). The development and maturation of the nervous system depends on extensive neural development processes that are shaped in a highly complex interaction that integrates and co-ordinates the neuroanatomical and neurobiological development with the relational contact to which the child has access in his or her close relations. In our view, it is precisely these specific interactions, which are such an essential aspect of the non-specific factor in child psychotherapy, that make it possible to develop the neural structures that provide the stimuli which the nervous system needs in order to initiate the process of personality development.


## Attachment experiences through the zone of proximal development

Stern (1995) has described that our self-image depends on the presence and actions of others, and that the child is drawn forwards in his or her development by the carer who interacts, now, with the future child. Vygotsky (1978) pointed out that the basic mechanisms for internalising higher psychological functions arise in the interaction and only become intrapsychological at a later time. As described in the previous chapter, the internalisation process takes place in what Vygotsky called the zone of proximal development, which he defined as those functions that have not matured but are in the process of maturing. What the child is currently able to do only with the carer's help, he or she will be able to do independently in the future. Thus, all the higher personality functions emerge as the result of social interaction. In asymmetrical relations, for example, teacher–student, therapist–client, etc., one has a responsibility for protecting and supporting the child or client in the zone that is outside his or her coping capacity. Some of the qualities that exist in a healthy carer–child relationship are also found in the healthy therapist–client contact.

Several developmental psychologists, including Daniel Stern, have described how an infant who is only a few days old is able to co-regulate with his or her carer. As social processes are inherently unpredictable, the infant has to be able to adapt in order to maintain the connection. The Norwegian psychologist, Stein Bråten (1993, 1998), says that the infant has a capacity for altercentric participation, meaning that the child has an ability to engage in social interactions by first paying attention to the other. Hafstad and Øvreeide (2007) have expressed this very movingly:

> When I show you that I see you, then you see me, for in my helpless-
> ness I need for you to see me ... Your face comes before my own,
> because I need to have access to it in order to become me. (p. 102)

From around the age of two years, language plays a crucial role in the child's ability to convey experiences. Although the child also expresses emotions and bodily impulses through play and other behaviour, language is the medium of dialogue. The better able the child is to convey experiences through language, the greater is his or her capacity for relating experiences with nuance and for being met with understanding. On every level of mental organisation, the child has experiences that have not yet been put into language. The integration of mental levels of organisation is important for the child, and if the relationship between carer and child does not allow for this, then one hopes it can be developed in a psychotherapy process where the child has the experience of being contained, understood, and acknowledged. All children need to feel that they are seen with their experiences, and to share these experiences through matching interaction experiences and narratives that are created in an intersubjective field. It is these present moments that we look for in child psychotherapy.

Before we look at MacLean's model of the triune brain and mental organisations, we want briefly to outline our view of the asymmetrical therapy alliance in the perspective of dynamic systemic theory, which regards the brain as a non-linear, self-organising system which develops through interactions with another non-linear, self-organising system. The asymmetrical alliance is comparable to the attunement that takes places in "healthy" carer–child relations, and the same attunement can be achieved in the therapeutic relationship. The only thing capable of healing inadequate attachment and ensuring personality development is the establishment of an attachment that is based on adaptive emotional attunement, which is undoubtedly the main reason behind the efficacy of psychotherapy in relation to relational disturbances and trauma healing.

## The brain as a self-organising system

In systemic theory, all development is based on self-organisation, and new, adapted forms of self-organisation develop from underlying components that enter into a complex hierarchical structure. As new capacities emerge, underlying components stabilise (Thelen, 1989). Neural patterns begin to form out of a multitude of components, and, in this process, the self-organising system becomes increasingly interconnected and organised. The many neural connections and combinations stabilise the nervous system and develop a growing capacity for maintaining permanence in relation to environmental variations.

As the nervous system develops, it comes to prefer a certain organisation and particular environmental context and tends towards previously established patterns. The stability of the system depends on its capacity for switching from one state to another. The nervous system develops in a self-organising process where one mental organisation is established on top of the preceding level. Every level of mental organisation builds on the previous level, and patterns of mental organisation are represented in hierarchical development. Changes happen in a non-linear fashion, and no one can predict the exact moment when the change is going to occur or the specific form development will take. Development represents a new element that is created in the self-organising process of the nervous system, which, in turn, can push the nervous system to a new state. Even tiny changes in self-organisation can lead to major changes in behaviour, which is what makes psychotherapy possible (Schore, 2003b; Siegel, 1999).

Although the brain is a self-organising system, it is also permeable and relies on external stimuli to develop. In connection with personality development, the stimulation and development of neural structures is mediated by the child's interactions with the primary carers and later with other significant others, including peers. It is this development potential that is the focus of the systematic psychotherapy process.

## The brain's emotional maturation processes

The maturation of the brain's emotional areas is crucial for determining which interactions the child invites and takes part in, and the response the child receives from the environment contributes to altering the neural structures. All higher personality functions, such as attachment capacity, emotional self-regulation, impulse control, and reflection, are acquired through countless social micro-interactions that are internalised and gradually develop the child's intrapsychological habits and structures. Since this process of learning and internalisation can only occur on the child's current level of maturation and within the child's zone of proximal development, therapists need to have insight into brain maturation and growth spurts. In children with normal functioning, the child's chronological age and the level of maturation are usually equivalent, but dysregulated and neglected children have a far more complex maturation process. For example, an eight-year-old boy might sometimes be in an age-appropriate zone of development with regard to his capacity for understanding requests and demands from adults, but display the emotional regulation capacity of a six-month-old infant when he is angry or startled. One of the non-specific factors in child therapy, therefore, is the therapist's ability to create interaction forms that satisfy the age-appropriate level of development as well as the child's immature development need.

In the following, we present a brief outline of the hierarchical brain and the three interrelated levels of mental organisation.

## The brain: a hierarchical and triune structure

Around 1900, Jackson (1958) pointed out that, over millions of years, the human brain has evolved "from the bottom up" and "from the inside out", as higher centres have emerged as superstructures to lower and older structures. He described the human brain as consisting of hierarchical functional levels where the functions at the top of the hierarchy are volitional and capable of inhibiting non-volitional, lower functions. In distinct development phases, the structures that develop early in life are progressively superseded by later-maturing structures, expanding the brain's complexity (Schore, 2003b). If functions in the top tiers of the hierarchy are damaged or impaired, lower functions will take over, as higher functions can only operate on the basis of lower functions, while lower functions can work independently of higher functions. The functions that were superior during early stages of development are gradually superseded by the higher and later-maturing levels and are regulated by them (Hart, 2008; Schore, 2003a,b).

In the late 1950s, MacLean (1990) developed his theory of the triune brain, which involves brain structures on three tiers that he considered quantum leaps in the evolution of the human brain. MacLean's concept of the brain as a hierarchical system is often used as a conceptual tool for understanding the hierarchical function of the brain (Figure 1).

He attributed the three brain structures with three forms of mentalization, with protomentalization as the most primitive, emotional mentalization as the middle level, and rational mentalization as the

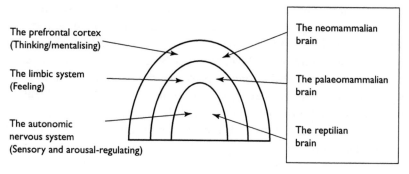

The prefrontal cortex
(Thinking/mentalising)

The limbic system
(Feeling)

The autonomic
nervous system
(Sensory and arousal-regulating)

The neomammalian
brain

The palaeomammalian
brain

The reptilian
brain

*Figure 1.*   MacLean's triune brain (source: Hart, 2011, p. 19).

third level. MacLean labelled the protomentalization, or autonomic sensory level, the reptilian brain. This section of the brain operates instinctively and consists of mid-brain structures and the brainstem, including the autonomic nervous system. Without the brainstem and the structures close to the brainstem and the autonomic nervous system, our nervous system would be unable to regulate arousal, and we would also be unable to sense emotions, because emotions and judgement are rooted in body sensations. Structures on this level are important for the child's capacity for spontaneous engagement with the world and for the functioning of the basic circuits for attention control, focusing, and presence in the moment (Damasio, 1999; Lewis, Amini, & Lannon, 2001).

In MacLean's taxonomy, the area of emotional mentalization is labelled the palaeomammalian brain, or the limbic system. The limbic system enabled the development and refinement of social interactions and, thus, also social emotions such as playfulness or sadness; it also added actual emotions to the brain's repertoire. The area of rational mentalization is called the neomammalian brain in MacLean's taxonomy.

This area processes cognitive rationales, and, among other functions, it enables us to mentalize, plan strategies, and maintain internal mental images (Hart, 2008).

## The triune brain and its mental organisations

In the 1980s, Chugani and colleagues (Chugani & Phelps, 1986; Chugani, Phelps, & Mazziotta, 1987) used PET-scans to measure the glucose metabolism in the infant brain. They discovered that the structures that were active at birth are relatively old evolutionary structures, while the brain structures that are activated later represent more recent evolutionary developments. Since this sequence of maturation defines the child's zone of proximal development and, in turn, which interactions are capable of promoting the child's maturation process, we shall take a closer look at this progression.

The higher up we go in the brain's hierarchical structures, the higher the degree of complexity. In the prefrontal cortex, the association network is highly developed and complex, and the greater the complexity, the greater is the potential that the psychological system can draw on to carry out sophisticated information processing of both emotional and cognitive content. Once the child's autonomic and limbic areas have matured, the child will engage in a narrative process to attempt to make sense of the world and to structure his or her own mental states. Sometimes, the narratives are also used for cognitive self-reflection. The human ability to reorganise our life stories lets us discover new ways of perceiving and experiencing our lives. The exchange of narratives reinforces and develops the brain's emotional and impulse-inhibiting structures, and it is through the process of narrative organisation that raw emotions are transformed into symbols. Verbal symbols make sense of the experience we acquire by feeling and perceiving. Through self-reflection, emotions are associated with an explicit understanding that might revise our narratives about who we are and build mentalized interpersonal connections. The condition for this process is an activation of the autonomic and limbic areas.

The brainstem, corresponding to the reptilian brain, is active from birth. Among other functions, it regulates arousal and sleep states and a wide variety of neurochemicals. This level of organisation activates and co-ordinates the organism's fundamental energy for interacting with the environment and regulates our affects and capacity for attention (Schore, 1994). At the age of two to three months, the visuospatial and motor functions begin to integrate, improving the child's ability to control his or her own movements based on emotions and pleasure-seeking impulses, which, in MacLean's evolutionary concept, corresponds to primitive mammals' motivation and levels of mental organisation. Eight months after birth, the last major brain area is activated: the frontal lobes, especially the prefrontal areas. These areas in particular enable us to develop the rational level of organisation, including some volitional control of our three levels of mental organisation. The three areas of mental organisation can be described as follows:

1.  The autonomic brain and the sensory level of organisation.
2.  The limbic brain and the emotional level of organisation.
3.  The prefrontal brain and the rationally mentalizing level of organisation.

The mental organisation levels do not develop in a linear fashion, but undergo critical maturation periods where they are particularly sensitive to the carers' capacity for interacting on the associated level of organisation, as they need this particular form of interaction to develop. As mentioned earlier, fundamental interactions with others is the dominant medium of emotional stimulation and, on early levels of development, this means interactions with the closest adult carers. The mental organisation on the three levels determines the nature of the moments of meeting and attunement processes that the child is capable of engaging in. This, in turn, defines three primary developmental forms of interaction that the carer has to be able to provide and engage in:

1. On the autonomic level, developmental interactions take place in the synchronised "dance" with the child's sensory impressions.
2. On the emotional level, developmental interactions take place in the attunement with the child's emotions.
3. On the mentalizing level, developmental interactions take place in a verbal dialogue with the child.

This development unfolds in the brain's first growth spurt, which begins *in utero* and ends around the age of two years. In Chapters Three, Four, and Five, we outline the normal development of the three levels and the naturally occurring interaction forms during the first growth spurt. In Chapter Six, we look at the continuing development of the mentalizing capacity during the second growth spurt, which begins around the age of two years and continues until adulthood.

## Interventions aimed at the triune brain

During the first two years of life, brain structures interconnect through huge neural circuits. Natural development involves an ongoing synchronisation among the various levels and areas, which means that all our experiences are based on reptilian-level sensations, mammalian-level emotions, and a conscious perception of context, verbally or non-verbally.

In Chapters Three, Four, and Five, in addition to introducing the mental organisations, we also present a model that adds further nuances to the three tiers of the triune brain and structures essential capacities and experiences on each of the levels: the neuroaffective compass model (Bentzen & Hart, 2012). We have developed a compass for each level of mental organisation, and the three compasses are seen as being interconnected, as illustrated in Figure 2. In each of the three chapters, we also describe one of the therapy forms and the associated case examples that were presented at the conference and identify non-specific factors on the given level of mental organisation, using the relevant compass. In Chapter Six, we describe the refinement of the prefrontal compass throughout the second growth spurt.

## Windows of opportunity

In the field of neuropsychology, it is well known that certain functions develop at certain times, depending on which area of the brain has a "window of opportunity", developmentally speaking. Hubel and Wiesel (1970) documented that kittens developed irreversible neural changes to their visual cortex when they were deprived of normal visual sensory impressions during a limited period of their early development. The same damage did not occur when the experiment was made on adult cats. The visual deprivation had an effect only when it occurred during the first three months of the kitten's life.

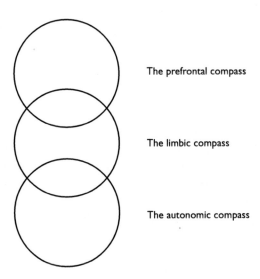

The prefrontal compass

The limbic compass

The autonomic compass

*Figure 2.*    The neuroaffective compasses (source: Bentzen & Hart, 2012, p. 107).

Thus, ideally, certain developments should take place at certain times, while the neural flexibility is high.

In most cases, the failure to acquire certain skills during sensitive periods is not irreversible, but some forms of learning are more reversible than others. A well-known example of a highly sensitive area is language acquisition. Regardless of how much language stimulation to which a six-month-old child is exposed, he or she will not be able to produce long grammatical sentences, because the neural conditions simply are not present at this stage. On the other hand, it is difficult to learn a new language and even harder to speak it without an accent after the age of approximately twelve years, unless the person has an innate talent for language. If a family with a four-year-old child, for example, moves to Spain, the child will be able to learn the language in less than six months simply by attending preschool daily, while the parents, despite attending work daily, will need language programmes to learn Spanish. Thus, the concept of "windows of opportunity" does not imply that the windows slam shut after a certain age, only that learning after this point requires a considerably more dedicated and deliberate effort. The same is true of the brain's emotional structures. There are indications that "windows of opportunity" for the basic emotional structures develop from the last trimester of pregnancy until around one year after birth. After this age, it takes a dedicated and deliberate effort to stimulate the basic emotional structures, which is the objective of most psychotherapy.

## "What works for whom?"

In their book *What Works for Whom?*, Roth and Fonagy (1996) note that the issue is not which therapeutic intervention is most effective but, rather, which form of intervention is of developmental benefit to whom. A variety of psychological treatment methods can lead to psychological development. Securely attached children and adults with a high mentalization capacity will probably have developed a sufficient degree of self-constancy to be able to engage with a narrative, dynamic, and interpretative treatment approach. Older children and adults who have developed a mentalization capacity will be able to symbolise and have fantasies, wishes, etc., that help organise self-regulation patterns and interactions with the therapist. Others who have not developed an adequate mentalization capacity undoubtedly will be unable to benefit from this psychological treatment approach and, instead, will require methods that are aimed more at attunement in the more deeply seated subcortical structures. Here, the emotional maturation involves building attention control, arousal regulation, affective attunement, etc., in order to elevate primitive pre-symbolic sensorimotor affects to mature symbolic representations. Fonagy (2005) even argues that some interventions might be harmful because they require capacities that the clients do not possess. This will only make them feel inadequate and might further exacerbate their condition.

It is necessary to meet the child in his or her zone of proximal development. For instance, a child who is on an immature level of organisation and has not yet developed sufficient capacity for play will not be able to take part in play therapy, where the child has to be able to externalise internal conflicts. An attempt at implementing this form of therapy might further disorganise the child's fragile nervous system. The intervention has to target areas where the child has developed some capacities and must be adjusted to match the child's level of mental organisation. In therapy with children with several relational disorders, it might, therefore, be necessary to use a "bottom-up" intervention in the form of autonomic and limbic attunement before moving on to methods that target higher levels of functioning. The same applies to the parents, who must also be met in their zone of proximal development.

Many psychological treatment methods take for granted that language can be used to effect change in profound affective processes in both the child and the parents. Most well-developed structured treatment methods often apply a narrative, symbolising approach. These methods are very well suited for families that have a mentalization capacity and will often be useful as brief interventions. However, in working with parents and children who have difficulties with arousal regulation and affective attunement, or who have a simplistic level of mentalization, there are few treatment methods to choose from, and they are always long term. We are convinced that if the given treatment method fails to target both the child's and the carers' zones of proximal development, there can be no present moments in the psychotherapy process, and, thus, the process will not be able to capture the non-specific factors that generate transformation. To achieve change, the method has to support the child in relation to his or her level of personality development. This means supporting the child in the areas where he or she seeks competence and coping and giving the child a chance to demonstrate independence in the areas where he or she has developed a capacity. It is important for the adult to attune with the child on all active levels of mental organisation.

Damage during early development can occur in three forms, as maturation potentials may be undeveloped, dissociated, or lost through regression. Finally, a maturation potential may also be over-developed and take on a compensatory function, as it serves as a proxy for other skills that are lacking. If the maturation potential is undeveloped, it will typically be possible only to stimulate it in a long-term targeted therapy process, because the neural circuits have failed to develop and, thus, need to be established at a time that lies outside their "windows of opportunity". In this case, the therapist has to act as a competent "caravan leader" who knows the way and who keeps the therapeutic work inside the boundaries of the child's zone of proximal development. Here, the focus is on enabling interactions with sensations, vitality affects, arousal regulation, and dyadic contact through shared focus and interest, repeated in new, but recognisable, ways until the child's experiences activate a new level of development. The next step is the development of internal experiences that can be represented symbolically and transformed in the context of play and its creative exploration of new possibilities, thus providing access to new action possibilities. Here, creative methods such as art therapy, play therapy, and sandplay, as well as methods with a cognitive behaviour focus, might prove highly effective.

## Child therapy in the perspective of neuroaffective developmental psychology

Before we move on to describing the specific mental organisations and compasses, we offer a brief outline of the psychotherapy process with children in the perspective of the hierarchical levels of mental organisation. When the emotional regulation is effective, the nervous system organises coherently, but when it fails, the brain's capacity for self-organisation and complex functioning is impaired, and it is often at this point that the child is referred to psychotherapy. Thus, although the effects of both misattunements and adaptive attunements reside in the child, resilience or deficiencies develop as a result of interactions with others. The emotional attunement between the child and the primary carer during the limbic period establishes the child's attachment pattern, which is crucial for the later capacity of the nervous system to engage in social relations and develop a mentalization capacity. The carer's ability to interpret and respond to the child's signals influences the child's stress modulation, and a child who feels secure will engage in explorative behaviour. Based on the model of mental organisations described above, psychotherapy should support the nervous system in three essential ways:

1.  Attunement on an autonomic level: supporting the child by activating curiosity, motor synchronisation, a musical variation between high-energy and calm, intimate activities, relaxation, perhaps being held and "contained within a field".
2.  Attunement on a limbic level: supporting the child through a focus on I–you, with emotionally marked mirroring, attunement, and dyadic, physical play with increasing arousal and pauses for "digesting" in the interactions.
3.  Attunement on a prefrontal level: together with the adults, the child verbalises how experiences and activities are experienced in the body in sensory and emotional terms. The adults support and affirm this process in a verbal dialogue.

Framed by the theory that is outlined above, the book *Neuroaffektiv psykoterapi med børn* (Hart, 2011) discusses some fundamental considerations in planning psychotherapy with a child. Here is a brief summary of these considerations:

•   the child needs to develop his or her emotional potential in an interaction that involves a symmetrical relationship with asymmetrical responsibility, where the person at the top of the power hierarchy has the full responsibility for providing leadership in a manner that trusts and acknowledges the child's experiences and feelings;
•   the child's symptoms or maladaptive behaviour reflect both innate capacities and a relational history that must be understood in full;
•   the child is only able to develop from his or her zone of proximal development; this means that the autonomic/sensory functions

and structures must develop prior to the limbic functions and structures; the limbic functions and structures must develop prior to the prefrontal ones, etc.;

- parents cannot support the development of those mental structures in their children that they have not themselves developed—"one cannot give what one does not possess".
- emotional development takes place through deep synchronisation processes and affective attunement.

## Summary

In this chapter, we have looked at the basis of neuroaffective developmental psychology and how this theoretical framework can produce a nuanced understanding of the non-specific factors in child psychotherapy. Psychotherapy is not only about calming the child's nervous system, but also about expanding the child's capacity for self-regulation and adaptive adjustment. Difficulties with arousal regulation and affect regulation are key elements in the child's symptom formations, and all child psychology treatment methods aim to develop the child's self-regulation capacity. Different psychological treatment methods target different areas in the hierarchical structure of the brain, and all forms of therapy seek to reintegrate and balance processes in the neural networks on different levels. The Russian psychologist, Lev Vygotsky, noted that development takes place in the child's zone of proximal development, which implies that the intervention needs to target the areas where the child has developed the beginnings of a capacity, and that the approach has to match the child's level of mental organisation.

The micro-regulatory interactions that unfold between carer and child normally occur within "windows of opportunity" in the child's zone of proximal development. To enable the micro-regulatory interactions that support the self-organisation of neural processes and the development of the self-regulation capacity, the therapy, therefore, has to challenge the nervous system in the child's zone of proximal development. When the stimulation has to take place outside these typical "windows of opportunity", it is applied in a systematic process where it is crucial to match the child's developmental capacity—the therapist needs to find the "carrier wave".

CHAPTER THREE

# The autonomic compass and somatic experiencing

"One little piece at a time, because each piece adds to the others. It's like a teeny little island in this sea of trauma and overwhelm, and then you find another little island, and then another, and another, and then these islands come together to form a mass of stability, of presence in the here-and-now, even though there's this storming all around"

(Peter Levine)

I n this and the following three chapters, we describe the individual levels of mental organisations and compasses and relate them to the therapy forms that most clearly target the given level of mentalization. In this chapter, we look at the autonomic level of mentalization and the compass related to the autonomic sensory level. We also describe Peter Levine's approach, "somatic experiencing", and review two therapy cases that he presented at the conference, with his comments and our own reflections from the perspective of the autonomic compass.

## The autonomic nervous system

The autonomic nervous system consists of two branches: the sym pathetic nervous system and the parasympathetic nervous system. The area is regulated reflexively, and the sympathetic and the parasympathetic nervous system have opposite functions. Normally, the autonomic nervous system varies between predominantly sympathetic and predominantly parasympathetic activation. The sympathetic nervous system activates motor activity such as rough-and-tumble play and fight-or-flight reactions. The parasympathetic nervous system normally activates rest states and vegetative functions, such as digestion and organ repair. In situations of immediate danger, where both fight and flight have proved ineffective or impossible, the parasympathetic nervous system activates either a motor block or freeze response, or motor collapse and surrender. If these autonomic self-protection responses are not terminated and turned off again once the danger has passed, the result will be a long-term shift in the autonomic balance towards either hyperactivity or passivity, which impairs the nervous system's capacity for regeneration and stress management (see Porges, 1998).

In the human brain, neural circuits associate facial expressions with brainstem activity, which means that facial mimicry and eye contact affect our breathing and heart rate. When an emotional state arises, it alters our heart rate, which, in turn, influences brain activity. Throughout life, we engage in sustained eye contact only in deep, emotional meetings of trust, intense rough-and-tumble play, and aggressive confrontations; sustained eye contact, therefore, has a highly activating sympathetic effect. Thus, when an adult demands that a dysregulated child maintain eye contact to prove that he or she is paying attention, the child will have considerable difficulty regulating his or her already shaky nervous system, and it is very likely that the child is unable to hear or understand the message.

Porges (1995, 1997, 1998) describes that the brain–body connection is mediated by the tenth cranial nerve, the vagus nerve (the wandering nerve). This nerve serves as a two-way link with many of the visceral organs, which means that it also provides feedback to the brain about the state of the body. The vagus nerve is connected to many of the body's internal organs, including the respiratory system, the heart, and the gastrointestinal system. The nervous fibres leading to the heart spring from two different branches of the nerve, which emerge in the lower section of the brainstem: the dorsal branch (nearest the back) and the ventral branch (nearest the front of the body). The dorsal branch is associated with biophysiological regulation and fight or flight, while the ventral branch is associated with psychobiological intersubjective regulation through its connection to the seventh cranial nerve. This facial cranial nerve arises close to the point where the ventral section of the vagus nerve has its roots, which is why caring and joy-filled communication through facial expressions can calm the heart.

Stimulating the muscles that activate facial mimicry thus promotes calm and self-regulation and ensures the potential for emotional attunement. The facial muscles influence both our emotional expressions and the impressions we form of others, and they can effectively reduce or increase the social distance. The neural regulation of the facial muscles serves both as an active social engagement system that reduces psychological distances and as a filter that influences our perception of other people's engagement behaviour (Hart & Kæreby, 2012; Porges, 2003).

## *The autonomic and sensory level of organisation*

The first level of mental organisation matures from the final trimester of pregnancy until around three months after birth. This level of mental organisation is associated with processes in the brainstem, mid-brain structures, and the autonomic nervous system. These areas regulate endocrine processes, immune reactions, digestion, breathing, heart rate, the secretion of neurochemicals, innate reflexes such as seeking, sucking, and grasping, and basic attention control. The infant's experiences of pleasure *vs.* displeasure in the carer's interactions with the infant's basic needs and autonomic processes form the basis for subsequent emotional experiences and assessments, which, in turn, shape the older child's thinking and behaviour. Simply put, the autonomic nervous system is the personality's physiological basis for sensing anything at all. Brainstem processes are responsible for our spontaneous engagement in the world, and the brainstem contains our basic circuits for attention control and intimacy (Damasio, 1999; Lewis, Amini, & Lannon, 2001).

The child's early sense of being alive comes from being physically active and receiving care. Touch and the development of the kinaesthetic sense play an important role as the child gradually senses his or her own boundaries and being-in-the-world. From birth, the infant is also, to some degree, able to perceive the world through all five sensory modalities: vision, hearing, smell, taste, and touch.

Stern has described internal body sensations, such as rush, crescendo, tension, liveliness, etc., as vitality affects. The infant already expresses these experiential modalities through movements and facial expressions during the first weeks of life and is able to express both pleasure and displeasure in relation to experiences. From the beginning of life, the child's experience of the world is influenced by the arousal of vitality affects, which help the infant navigate in the world. To develop a sense of being-in-the-world, the infant needs recurring proprioceptive experiences as well as experiences with internal patterns of tension and vitality affects (Stern, 1985). Neglect or traumatic experiences can, however, lead to underdeveloped, impaired, or dissociated body sensations and vitality affects, which will cause these basic functions to be damaged and disturbed.

In child psychotherapy and interventions, interactions on the autonomic level of mentalization are crucial, as this is the level where all experiences of moments of meeting and intersubjective synchronisation, and, thus, all personal learning, happen and are integrated. Play and physical activity are commonly included in interventions with children, but to support the autonomic maturation process the bodily attention needs to be linked with the innate capacity for synchronising with others through arousal-regulating and emotional interactions.

The child's capacity for imitation enables the child to copy subtle physical reactions as reflected in the carer's facial expression from one moment to the next and, thus, attune with these reactions. The child imitates the carer's postures, facial expressions, and prosody, and deep-seated areas in the brain mediate the association of imitation and bodily sensations with the carer's attuned support. By synchronising with the carer's state through imitation and bodily sensations, the child develops a sense of the adult's emotional state, the precursor of empathy. This internal mirroring makes the interaction interesting, thus triggering curiosity and developing the child's capacity for sustained engagement. Thus, if the child has lacked opportunities for imitative contact with carers during the first months of life, the seeds will have been sown for a profound disturbance of attention control, the deepest layers of the attachment processes, and the development of empathy.

The infant possesses only limited means for regulating his or her mental state and, therefore, often withdraws from stimulation that feels too intense. For example, during a positive interaction the child might withdraw in order to dampen his or her emotional excitement and then resume the interaction after a break. The infant also seeks soothing and arousal regulation by sucking on his or her thumb or a dummy/pacifier. Crying, vocalisation, and smiles help the infant present him/herself as a social individual who is capable of engaging social interactions and who responds emotionally to events. The infant's spontaneous facial expressions and crying also trigger a response in the carer, who assigns specific meaning to these expressions, and the carer's responses contribute to the growing sophistication of the infant's inner world (Emde, 1992; Sroufe, 1996).

## The autonomic compass

The autonomic compass is a model of the individual's energy management and body sensations. The compass is structured around two axes: the axis of arousal regulation, which relates to sympathetic and parasympathetic activity, and the axis of hedonic tone, which relates to the sensation of pleasure and displeasure (Figure 3).

Arousal regulation is crucial for psychological resilience and is, therefore, a key element in psychotherapy and other forms of treatment. Activation of the sympathetic nervous system creates a reflexive focus of attention with a deep sensory awareness and motor preparedness, while the activation of the calming system (the parasympathetic nervous system) creates a relaxed state. The variation between the two poles increases the child's response capacity and helps develop self-protection strategies against stimulus overload and stress (Hart, 2008, 2010). Both sympathetic activation and parasympathetic down-regulation are normally accompanied by a specific hedonic tone, which means that they are perceived as either pleasant or unpleasant. As Peter Levine said (private communication, 2009), this ability to distinguish between pleasant and unpleasant draws on

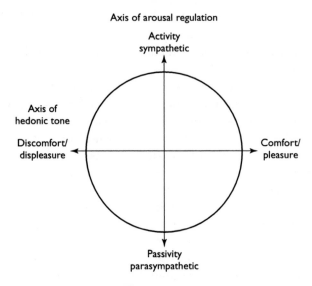

*Figure 3.* The autonomic compass.

basic levels of cellular functioning, but it may be lost or underdeveloped in the case of early neglect/abuse and in dissociative states.

Combining the axis of arousal regulation and the hedonic axis produces four quadrants that cover the basic forms of experience on the brainstem level. From everyday activities and experiences, we are familiar with the pleasant (hedonic) experience of sympathetic activity, which is associated with such activities as play and sport, and which can produce a feeling of excitement and vitality, while the parasympathetic state feels calm and relaxed. The unpleasant (dyshedonic) experience of sympathetic activity includes experiences of vigilance, watchfulness, defensiveness, and fight-or-flight responses, while the unpleasant parasympathetic experience is one of apathy, indifference, sudden freeze, or immobilisation (Figure 4). All these states occur naturally, and most people will have experienced more or less pronounced versions of most of these states. The healthy position, thus, involves a self-regulation capacity that is present in all the states. Psychological resilience implies that the optimal arousal zone is large, meaning that one is able to contain and manage both high- and low-intensity input and has a well-regulated capacity for varying between sympathetic and parasympathetic activity and for containing both pleasant and unpleasant states in a field of contact.

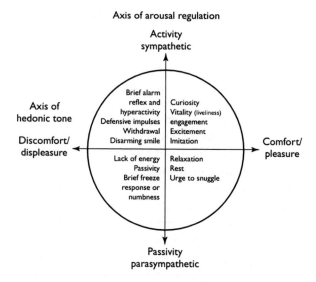

*Figure 4.*   The autonomic compass with interaction quadrants
(source: Bentzen & Hart, 2013, p. 65).

## The autonomic interaction quadrants

The regulation of both hedonic tone and arousal develops through regulated interactions in asymmetrical relations, that is, through attuned interactions with the carers based on activities that gradually increase parasympathetic and sympathetic activity in a way that maintains the synchronisation between the child's and the carer's nervous systems. The child's experiences of being able to maintain the contact with the carer stem initially from pleasant experiences and later develop to include the ability to maintain contact in high- or low-arousal unpleasant experiences, which contributes to the maturation of self-regulating strategies on this level. An older child who has developed a self-regulation capacity regulates flexibly in and out of these states in an ongoing interaction with the potentials and possible dangers of the moment.

The more vulnerable the nervous system, the greater caution one has to display in increasing sympathetic and parasympathetic activity and the dyshedonic state. This applies both to the carer's contact with the infant and to the therapeutic contact; when the child is able to develop and maintain the regulating interactions with the world, he or she develops resilience.

## Autonomic self-protection strategies

As mentioned above, the "healthy" nervous system that has developed a self-regulation capacity will regulate flexibly in and out of the states described above in an ongoing interaction with the possibilities and potential dangers that are present in the environment at any given moment. However, the nervous system may also get stuck in one of these four states as a self-protection strategy, or flutter between them without balance. An extreme version of the pleasant sympathetic quadrant is the child who becomes over-excited in a manic state or "rush" to expend energy. An extreme version of the pleasant parasympathetic quadrant might be addiction to television watching or hiding in one's room for long periods without any contact to the outside world. The unbalanced unpleasant sympathetic state might be characterised by severe startle responses, stressful or traumatic hyperactivity, or unmotivated fight-or-flight responses. Finally, there is the extreme version of the unpleasant parasympathetic state, which is evident as dissociation, frozen physical immobilisation or paralysis, or the loss of feelings and a capacity for contact with others (Figure 5). All these states reflect a loss of the capacity to engage in synchronised interactions with significant others.

In more severe cases, we see a chronic fixation in the dyshedonic state from an early age: for example, in a reactive attachment disorder, which can either leave the person fixated in immobilisation, fixated in the fight or flight state, or switching back and forth between the two. The fixation implies a loss of a proprioceptive qualitative experience (the person feels neither comfort nor discomfort) and the ability to engage in synchronised interactions. The inability to regulate out of comfort and discomfort implies severe difficulties with arousal regulation. In addition, the personality is locked into the autonomic sensory level, where one cannot understand one's own share in events but is limited to primitive projections; other people are perceived as unpredictable, and there is no trust of their intentions. This state is often characterised as reactive attachment disorder, sociopathy, or other personality disorder.

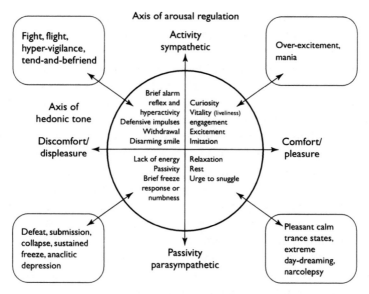

*Figure 5.*  The autonomic compass with self-protection strategies
(source: Bentzen & Hart, 2013, p. 67)

## Child psychotherapy and balancing the autonomic compass

In the therapeutic relationship, the therapist's arousal regulation capacity on the level of the autonomic nervous system and the therapist's capacity for maintaining contact with the child's autonomic nervous system become the source of the child's development of a self-regulation capacity.

An optimal psychotherapeutic effort on this level involves engaging with the child's autonomic nervous system in order to resolve fixations in the autonomic nervous system. Together with the child, the therapist moves in soft, rhythmic waves of activation in a process resembling a dance that varies between sympathetic and parasympathetic activation and between pleasant and unpleasant states. When working with unpleasant states, the child benefits from the interaction with the therapist's calm autonomic nervous system and experiences the possibility of returning from an unpleasant internal experience to a pleasant one. This is a direct coping experience, beyond words, that makes it less overwhelming to approach the unpleasant state to explore it further. Enhanced coping skills in the "landscape" of arousal regulation improve the capacity for self-organisation or resilience on

the level of the autonomic nervous system. It is typically more difficult to work with the hedonically pleasant self-protection strategies,
such as fidgeting, as they often border on an addiction which can be
so compelling that it can be difficult to bring the child into a field of
contact. However, the first step is still to let the nervous system
discover that it has other options; that it may, for example, move from
a dazed, dream-like, introvert state to a pleasant, or even slightly
exciting, activity. When working with over-excited hyperactivity, the
key is to test how far down in arousal it might feel pleasant to go
before the self-protection impulse drives the activity level up again.
At this stage, therapy is about building experiences that demonstrate satisfactory alternative experiences to the active self-protection
strategy. As the number of these alternative experiences increases,
the autonomic nervous system will often switch spontaneously to a
healthier self-regulating rhythm at some point. These are just a few of
the guidelines for the dance of attunement that should unfold in the
field of contact in the autonomic nervous system.

Self-protection strategies from the autonomic and sensory level of
organisation play a particularly prominent role in connection with
neglect, abuse, and trauma disorders. However, it is only in recent
decades, with the growing understanding of post traumatic stress
disorder (PTSD) in adults, that the autonomic level has begun to be
included in psychotherapy, and there are still only very few treatment
methods for children that address the regulatory forms of interactions
on this basic level of mentalization. However, Peter Levine, the creator
of the somatic experiencing therapy, has developed a therapeutic
theory and method that has been used especially in trauma therapy,
and which aims specifically at regulation and improved functioning
on this level (Levine, 1983; Levine & Kline, 2006, 2009) by supporting
the traumatised person in completing bodily self-protection strategies
and establishing a sense of mastery in his or her own body. Since all
interpersonal development and intrapsychological regulation depend
on this level, we consider it essential for therapists to have both a
theoretical understanding and practical intervention methods that can
help children learn to regulate on this level. In the following section,
therefore, we look at the earliest development of a proto-level of
mentalization in order to gain an understanding of some of the subtle
intersubjective synchronised dances that form the core of regulation
efforts on this level.

### Dancing with the autonomic compass:
### a presentation of somatic experiencing by Peter Levine

Peter Levine has spent more than forty years exploring the autonomic nervous system's self-regulation in states of rest, healthy activation, stressful states, and post traumatic stress. Against this background, he has developed psychotherapeutic interactions and methods to help regulate the autonomic nervous system and assist in developing an improved capacity for regulation and resilience. Much of this work has involved adults suffering from severe traumatisation, but, since the method is not dependent on language, Peter Levine has also worked for decades with children, even very young children, ranging from newly born to eighteen years of age.

Somatic experiencing rests on two main pillars: one is to regulate affective and sensorimotor states in the framework of the therapeutic relationship, and the other is to teach the child self-regulation skills by deliberately and attentively contacting, following, and, in older children and adults, helping to verbalise sensorimotor processes. This helps to restore and develop the child's social engagement system and to integrate intense experiences, sensorimotor reactions, and arousal states. Engaged presence is the key therapeutic vehicle for making the child more aware of internal sensorimotor reactions and strengthening his or her capacity for self-regulation. The purpose of somatic experiencing is to give the child tools for handling disturbing bodily reactions and being able to process them both emotionally and cognitively.

Levine describes nine steps in the psychotherapeutic method of somatic experiencing.

1.  The therapist must first establish an environment of *relative safety* in the room and in the interaction.
2.  Next, the therapist works with the child to begin the initial *exploration and acceptance of sensation*. This creates a resource experience in the therapeutic contact.
3.  Now, the therapist works with the child to gradually establish the natural autonomic movement between the stressful state and the resource experience, between high and low arousal, until the child feels safe in this movement. This rhythmic movement is called *pendulation*.

4.  The therapist now includes the more intense arousal states, making sure that the child only briefly touches them, and actively guides the child into long integration periods in between each of these brief experiences. This aspect is called *containment*.

5.  The containment process is followed by *titration*, which means that the therapist gradually, drop by drop, adds increasingly survival-based arousal and other challenging sensory experiences *in the rhythm and with the degree of challenge that the nervous system is able to integrate through pendulation*. This process leads to increasing stability, resilience, and structure in the autonomic regulation.

6.  The therapist now offers the child corrective experiences to supplant the passive autonomic reaction patterns of collapse and helplessness. The therapist does this by inviting or supporting the child's exploration of active empowered defensive responses while continuing the containing activity to prevent the child and the environment from being injured or overwhelmed.

7.  The therapist identifies the acquired association between fear and helplessness, on the one hand, and the biological immobility response, on the other, and facilitates a separation or "uncoupling" of the two states. This enables the child to feel scared and helpless without entering immobility.

8.  Only now does the therapist attempt to resolve states of hyperarousal by gently guiding the discharge and the redistribution of the huge amount of survival energy that the child mobilised in order to survive. This can be done, for example, in a safe physical exploration of the many ways in which it is possible to fall down without getting hurt, or through a slow-motion exploration of the strength in the falling reflexes of the arms when working with the after-effects of a bicycle crash. When the survival impulses are integrated, this energy is released in support of more highly developed mental functions.

9.  The self-regulation capacities are restored, in part through an accepting and attentive process of staying with sensations, feelings, and bodily impulses, orientating towards the "here and now" and an ability to reconnect with the environment along with a capacity for social engagement.

In every step of this process, the therapist makes sure to keep the child's arousal levels within the optimal zone of arousal, as described in the four quadrants of the autonomic compass. In traumatic reactions, the arousal typically increases initially, until it exceeds the optimal limit, which warns the person of a potential threat. In successful and energised fight-or-flight responses, this high arousal is utilised in physical activity with the purpose of defending and restoring the organismic balance. If the child's arousal can express itself optimally in this way, the level returns to the optimal zone. A failure to return to baseline is a key factor in the problems of hyperarousal that characterise the traumatised child.

A key insight in somatic experiencing is that when arousal is kept within the optimal zone, both children and adults are able to process information efficiently, which means that they are able to experience internal reactions without dissociating from the affects, sensations, sensory perceptions, and thoughts that come up.

After this brief introduction to Peter Levine's therapeutic method, we now turn to his conference presentation of sessions with children.

## Video clips from somatic experiencing sessions presented at the conference by Peter Levine

### Therapy with Simon

Peter Levine's first demonstration video dealt with fourteen-month-old Simon, who had been born in a dramatic emergency caesarean. We give the floor to Peter Levine.

> At birth, Simon had the umbilical cord three times around his neck. The doctors performed an emergency caesarean because there was a very strong heart rate deceleration, but they still couldn't get him out because he was breeched. His head was wedged in on the apex against the diaphragm, so they had to suction him out, and then he went into intensive care—all kinds of tubes and pin-pricks and so forth. And when you see Simon, he really appears and *is* a relatively normal child, but he doesn't really mould, attach, snuggle with his mother— he doesn't have that capacity. He's a very bright child, in many ways, aware of what's going on in the environment, but he doesn't share that with the parents. The mother is very clearly, at least in Winnicott's terms, a "good-enough" mother. There isn't anything that she is doing that limits his capacity.

The reason I'm seeing him is he has choking and gastric reflux. They are very concerned about this, and so they want to do an endoscopy of the lungs and the oesophagus and the stomach. And this, as you can imagine, is extremely traumatic. So I'm hoping to see if I can reverse this. Normally with a child, I'll start playing and then gradually get to know them and work with what's going on, but with Simon I come in much more quickly than I normally would.

At fourteen months, of course, he has very little language, so the question is, how do I interact with him, how do I connect with him, how do I see where the problem is, and how do I help him to transform that problem? Think of the situation again: being stuck in the birth canal, trying to push your way out, the more you push, the more you get stuck. The response to that is to resign, to go helpless, especially because, again, he's pulled out, so his agency really is not engaged.

Here, Peter Levine described reaction patterns from the autonomic nervous system. Studies of children just after birth have found that the catecholamine level and, thus, sympathetic activation is several times higher than normal. Levine explained that as the perceived life threat persisted and was even intensified, Simon's parasympathetic surrender response would have taken over. As a result, fourteen months later, Simon had not yet attuned with his mother. Based on Simon's history and his symptoms, the problem appeared to be on a physio-biological level, as Simon did not display the mammalian cub's innate snuggle reflex and, in addition, had eating difficulties and problems with gastric reflux, which would normally have been regulated by his synchronisation with his mother. The gastric reflux problem suggests a very high stress level, where Simon's autonomic self-protection strategies had become stuck in a freeze response, which also meant that the sympathetic fight-or-flight reactions were highly activated, while the parasympathetic brake blocked any motor activity. In terms of the autonomic compass, Simon was in the dissociated field, where a highly dyshedonic tone was associated with parasympathetic arousal but combined with an underlying negatively charged sympathetic arousal.

Peter Levine continued:

First of all, I try to establish a connection with Simon through rhythmicity. This is a key point, a key variable, and I think that you have maybe one minute to establish that, to really connect and to see the problem. Next, you can guide the person in what will restore the sense of agency and capacity for connectedness. What I'm looking for is the beginning of his capacity to defend himself, as his basic experience is being in a passive situation, and whatever he does has no positive effect on his feeling of okayness, goodness, safety. Then I have to follow the charge in his body as he starts to be able to defend himself, and the amazing thing is that no matter how overwhelmed we are, there exists in us a latent capacity to rebound from this overwhelm and to return to a state of vitality and curiosity and engagement. But we have to observe where the impulses have been stuck and then to support their emergence to re-establish the organising capacity.

*The video begins. We see Simon sitting on his mother's arm, facing away from Peter Levine, who is standing about two feet away, trying to get his attention with a rattle that he is shaking close to Simon's hand. Simon gives Levine a brief glance and then withdraws his hand.*

Peter Levine described the sequence in the recording:

First step: Simon withdraws his arm—this is not approach, this is not curiosity, this is into the negative hedonic region.

*Simon turns to look at Peter Levine and the rattle again.*

He still has a little curiosity . . .

*Simon pushes the rattle away and turns to face the mother.*

That's the first time he pushes away. There is an engagement that allows that impulse to unfold. So, in some way, there's a structure to what we're doing, because we first establish a rhythmicity, then we seek engagement, and then we activate our self-protection impulses. But at the same time, psychotherapy really is unstructured, because we're looking for what emerges.

*Peter Levine continues contacting Simon with a compassionate and soothing "Ah yeah, yeah, yeah . . ." The mother turns away slightly, shielding Simon, who is squirming and spinning. Peter Levine says to him, encouragingly, "Ah, you're spinning, huh?"*

So here we have the vestibular, the cerebellar, the sound of rhythm, movement, all of this has the effect of helping him modulate his nervous system response. Each time he has these experiences, where the rhythm, his movement, and my response form a coherent experience, what Susan and Marianne called micro-regulations, his experience of the world is altered. Instead of experiencing it as alien and threatening, he experiences it as engaging and curiosity-invoking.

*Peter Levine says to Simon, "You're a spinner," and the mother replied, "He's a spinner!" In a gentle, compassionate tone, Levine says to Simon, "Boy, you had quite a difficult time, didn't you, getting into this world." The mother answered, "He did, he did." Simon turns and almost faces Levine, then points past him and says, "Apple!"*

And now he sees something; again, the curiosity: "Apple", there's something in his environment. It turns out, by the way, that it's not an apple, it's a pomegranate; in fact it's three pomegranates in a bowl on the table. He sees it, and he wants to have something to do with it. So again, when the defence response is re-established—boom, the curiosity re-emerges.

*In the video, Simon touches the pomegranate and then pushes it away. His mother says, "Yeah, that's okay." Peter Levine answers, "Actually, with all those tubes and all those kind of things, I can see why he'd want to push things away . . ."*

Here we see curiosity and defence response. Each of those is critical. Without them, the work that I do would be impossible.

In this sequence, Peter Levine worked with Simon to establish a rhythm between curiosity and the defensive response, which belong in the two sympathetic arousal quadrants in the autonomic compass. The interaction was interspersed with breaks where Peter Levine talked to Simon or the mother. Peter Levine offered organising experiences in the form of the rattle and the pomegranates, and he noticed and supported even the smallest indications from Simon to determine whether the next interaction should aim at curiosity, self-protection, or a pause. At the same time, the mother was fully engaged in this guiding process, which allowed Simon's nervous system to exchange with and be regulated by two secure and precisely attuned adult nervous systems.

*In the video, the mother makes supportive, encouraging cooing noises: "Yeah, yeah". Simon makes a little hiccuppy sound, and the mother says, "Ooh, sweetheart." Peter Levine invites Simon and the mother to sit on the sofa. Simon whimpers a little and begins to kick off his shoes. Peter Levine says, "Bye-bye! Bye-bye, shoes" and the mother joins in: "Bye-bye, shoes!" Then, Peter Levine begins to discuss the forthcoming endoscopy with the mother.*

I see Simon stiffen as we start talking about the surgery. I'm not saying that this is caused by the topic of our conversation, but I see that he stiffens, particularly in the mid-dorsal, which is something I've observed in many different situations. This area of the body is very important in regulating the peristalsis, and in some of the early osteopathic literature this is considered a reflex point.

*In the video, the mother and Peter Levine talk about the problem with gastric reflux while Simon and the mother are sitting face-to-face. When Peter Levine reaches out to touch Simon in the middle of his back, Simon pushes him away and whimpers slightly.*

There! You see that; that's a key, when Simon pushes away with his legs, which is what was thwarted in the birth process. So each time this impulse emerges, he comes out of the passivity and shut-down and into an active engagement. One little piece at a time, because each piece adds to the others. It's like a teeny little island in this sea of trauma and overwhelm, and then you find another little island, and then another, and another, and then these islands come together to form a mass of stability, of presence in the here-and-now, even though there's this storming all around.

*In the video, Simon whimpers slightly, and the mother laughs gently. Peter Levine says, with compassion, "Oh, sweetie, yeah, ooh . . ." and the mother continues to explain the reflux problem.*

Again, when she's talking about the problem, I'm not saying that he understands that, but his body understands something.

*In the video, the mother speaks about the trauma, and Simon pushes away with his legs. Peter Levine replies, "Yeah, yeah, yeah, that's a touchy area, huh? I wish we had more time to play, but since you're having this procedure, it'd be nice if you don't have to have the procedure. Yeah, you're pushing me away, yeah."*

And again, it's stronger, the pushing is stronger every time, it's building, he's starting to restore the capacity he had lost.

*In the video, Simon cries, and Peter Levine says, "Yeah, it's okay; you can push me, yeah, oh . . ."*

It's a collapse, but it's also a discharge, it's a releasing. And the mother says in a moment that she's never heard or seen him cry like this, she's never seen tears."

*In the video, Simon cries louder, and Peter Levine says, "Atta boy, yeah, that's a boy. Yeah, you had all kinds of people touching you in not such nice ways." Simon is crying deeper now, the breath comes through in stronger rhythms.*

And you see there; he's crying but he's also staying in contact with me. This is another key aspect: to be able to be in a distress state but to stay in contact.

*In the video, Peter Levine says to Simon, "Having a good cry, yeah" and to the mother, "This area I was touching, it's very touchy, he doesn't want it. He's very tight there." The mother says, "I was just about to say, he never cries," and Levine replied, "Yeah, I was about to ask you, because to me this looks like a very emotional release."*

But really, Simon *does* want me to touch him, he's accepting it now. And if you listen to the frequencies now, there are frequencies that are like the ones you hear in the birth cries.

*In the video, Peter Levine says, "And that needs to happen." Simon is crying, and Levine comments: "Yeah, we really got that place, huh?"*

Now, this is wonderful, you see, I'm kind of in his face. He doesn't like that.

*In the video, Peter Levine wags his index finger close to Simon's face; Simon pushes him away very assertively.*

Now he's sort of playing with his power. He's crying, but he's also playing with his power. You see the mother's face, it's like she's saying, "I'm not sure what to do with this. Like, oh my god, this is my child?!" The problem was not there because she's a bad mother, not at all. The problem was that Simon's life energy, his core regulation, was derailed right at the beginning. And when that comes into balance, you see so many things start to fall into place.

*In the video, the mother says, "Oh, he's really hot!"*

She's feeling the discharge, heat, vasodilation, a very strong autonomic shift, and *now* he settles.

*Simon's crying dissipates into deep gasps and breaths.*

And this is the sequence of defensive responses: the shaking and trembling, the heat and then the breath. This is the language of the autonomic nervous system.

*In the video, Simon gives a deep sigh. Peter Levine says to the mother, "Did you hear that breath!" Finally, Simon buries his head in his mother's shoulder.*

As the core system comes into alignment, then the developmental stages in this case are falling into place. Now he just innately, instinctively wants to mould, wants to approach, wants to be held, wants to be soothed.

*In the video, the mother gently rocks back and forth, while Simon whimpers a little, relaxing. The mother put her hand on Simon's back, and Peter Levine says, "Good, let's wait and see, I don't want to do any more right now, I think this is just the right amount right now, especially since he had such a strong reaction, very uncharacteristic" and the mother replies, "Yeah, I've never seen, even when he gets frustrated, he's not . . . Did he go to sleep?!"*

The mother is not quite sure if he's asleep, she is just now learning her own sensations of attachment. Simon is kind of looking around, noticing if my hand gets close enough again—he's probably going to bite it off! And now, there's that smile, like he's saying, "What's this guy about?!" The mother says he never does this; he'll touch, and then he'll move on to the next thing. If this had not been renegotiated, this is something that probably would have played out in his different relationships. And in his health.

*In the video, Peter Levine says, "What a smile! Hi, Simon!" Simon's mother comments, "This is very . . . He's very affectionate, but he's not still, unless he's sleeping. By himself he's very peaceful, you know, he'll be still, but if there's other people and they're touching or stroking or . . ." She is clearly deeply emotionally affected by what she is seeing in her son. Peter Levine says to Simon, "Yeah, you've got a lot a stuff you're working through there, yeah." Simon looks assertive and tucks his hand away. He maintains eye contact with Peter Levine and smiles, clearly feeling secure, while his mother rocks gently. Simon is able to look away, withdraw, and then re-establish eye contact with Peter Levine.*

### Second session, one week later

*In the video, the mother explains that she has been taking notes about Simon, and she says, "Probably one of the biggest things was that at 1.30 that night after we were here, he woke up, which isn't normal for him . . . and he didn't cry, but he called out 'mama', and I went to get him, and he wanted to do this . . ." [shows snuggle motion], ". . . and then was patting me for a little bit, and then he said 'apple'; and I thought he wanted to eat, but he wanted this." The mother smiles and points to the pomegranate.*

> Simon wanted to come back. Mum had taken him back to the paediatric surgeon—and Simon obviously had sensed that this is not something that he wanted to have happen—so when they were leaving, and they're driving in the car, he says "pizza", and mum says, "oh, you want some pizza", and he said, "no, apple."

*In the video, Simon looks around curiously, and the mother says to Peter Levine, "So this is not him; I mean, this is the new him!" Levine replies, "Can you give me one example of what he's been like?" and the mother replies, "He's been really good, I mean, he's been sick, he had a cold, but he's been much more talkative, much more interactive with us, wants to show us a lot of things, he wants our feedback more. This is . . . I can't tell you . . . he's always been a very affectionate kid, but to just want to sit here and be cuddled in is a complete change, I mean it's wonderful for me, it's just totally unlike the way that he was before." Meanwhile, Simon is looking around, active and taking everything in.*

> In a sense, this is a very simple intervention—what it requires, though, is paying attention . . ."

Peter Levine looks at the conference audience, many of whom are tearing up and sniffling slightly.

> How are you all doing? I mean, we all were infants, we all were born, we all had mothers, so, how are you all doing . . . OK? Just being with these sensations and feelings, whatever they are . . . And just as Susan and Marianne described, these micro-regulations just seep from one into the other into the other, and you see this macro-unfolding, but the key is in the micro-expressions.

### Therapy with Johnny and Susie

In the following, we describe excerpts from Peter Levine's second demonstration video, which involved an intervention with Johnny and his big sister Susie. A few months earlier, two-year-old Johnny had fallen through the plastic tarpaulin covering the family's outdoor whirlpool bath and become trapped underneath. Susie, who was not quite five yet, had found him like that and had run in to get her mother, who pulled him out of the water. Although the body was clinically dead, Johnny was resuscitated. After this incident, he had begun to wake up at night screaming, although he otherwise seemed to be a normal, healthy child. Susie, too, had had a bad shock. Her symptom was that if Johnny was out of her sight for a minute she would panic and run around in the house to look for him.

> *In the video, we see Johnny rocking energetically in a rocking chair in Peter Levine's consultation, while Levine's large, friendly dog, Pouncer, is moving around, wagging his tail. Levine is speaking with Susie, who was focused on watching herself on the video monitor. Peter Levine asks Susie what had happened when Johnny nearly drowned: "Do you remember?" Susie is making faces at the camera.*

> I've got her hooked! So now I can get back to Johnny. What we see here right at the beginning is vestibular stimulation from the movements of the rocking chair.

Peter Levine described characteristic self-soothing in the autonomic nervous system, the use of rocking to decrease stress and sympathetic arousal by affecting the vestibular system and vermis deep inside the cerebellum. However, the rocking motion is only a really effective means of self-soothing when it has been internalised through secure interactions with the carer. Rapid, jerky, and stereotyped rocking, as we saw with Johnny in the video, is often an attempt at diminishing stress or the unresolved internal discomfort of sustained dysregulation. Stereotyped movements can reduce the internal autonomic stress level slightly, but will not fully soothe the child.

*In the video, Susie describes how she found Johnny lying in the water; Johnny pays close attention to her story, and his legs immediately stiffen in the rocking chair. Susie demonstrates to Peter Levine how she stepped into the pool, and he asks her, "Can you show me how?" Johnny walks over to Susie and Peter Levine and steps up on the edge of the imaginary pool, which is the sofa with a mattress on the floor. Susie makes swimming strokes in the air while watching herself on the video monitor.*

When I saw Johnny's leg stiffen, that told me I had to be ready to help him elongate and restore his active defensive response. Most likely, his defensive response was to kick. So we want to re-establish that active response. And then Susie began to swim for him . . .

*In the video, Peter Levine says to Johnny, "And then you went in? Yeah, I bet that was a surprise to you? Suddenly you're in. Can you show me how? You put your foot in. Then what happened?" Johnny mimics blowing motions as he lets himself slide down the sofa on to the mattress with Peter Levine supporting him all the way down. Johnny lies on his stomach for a moment and then raises his head and an arm, as if he is trying to get out of the water.*

There it is: another defensive response: blowing the water out in micro-regulations—in micro-expressions. And then comes his attempt at getting out.

*In the video, Johnny is making swimming motions on the mattress; he says, "I do that!" Peter Levine replies, "Yeah, you were under the water doing that!" The mother, who is also present, says, "They're so happy to be together." Levine then says to Susie, "Yeah, I bet you are, I bet you're happy he's okay." The mother says to Susie, "Susie, can you tell Peter what happened to you?" Susie replies, "I got to go get a toy from the hospital." The mother laughs, shaking her head slightly, and Levine comments, "So is that what you remember the most, well that's good, you remember the nice part."*

It's important to know that just reinforcing the nice part is also a marker that he's still alive, that he didn't die. So what she needs to face in this renegotiation, this play, is when she thought he was dead. So we're gradually bringing her towards this.

*In the video, Johnny begins to bang on a drum while he watches Peter Levine. Levine comes over and suggests a way of hitting the drum, but Johnny picks up the drum . . . and goes on banging on it, BANG BANG BANG!*

Johnny's saying, 'I'll do it my way! Thanks for the suggestion, but no thanks!' So basically, now, I can relax, he takes care of things.

In the spontaneous arousal fluctuations in the autonomic compass, Peter Levine has now helped Johnny experience the small bodily memory segments of the terrifying fall into the whirlpool and the experience of being trapped under water, but in ways that are always supportive of sympathetic motor responses in the present and, thus, offer a sense of mastery. The drumming sequence is a high point in Johnny's experience of forceful and energised activity, linked to an age-appropriate prefrontal joy of coping, making one's own decisions, and challenging adult authority; Peter Levine supports his initiative. He consistently enhances both children's sense of mastery and talks about the events in a kind, empathic, and down-to-earth language in a manner that exemplifies the adult carer's marked mirroring, which is discussed in the next chapter; the marked mirroring that makes it possible for Johnny and Susie to integrate the scary memory in rough-and-tumble play.

*In the video, Peter Levine asks Susie how she thinks Johnny might have fallen in. "He was on his face flat like that." Pouncer is agitated and goes over to the children. Johnny mimics falling into water by falling off the sofa, "prac-tising" falling backwards. He and Susie begin to play a game of falling off the sofa on to the mattress below in many different ways.*

Now, both Johnny and Susie are starting to be a little bit more exuber-ant. They're starting to move from the very narrow and cautious repe-tition and transition towards more exuberance. Also, it's not important which way he actually fell, it's just practising all the differ-ent possibilities that could occur. By playing with the dangerous fall, he is developing resilience in relation to future situations that might be overwhelming. Afterwards, Johnny needs some space, so he leaves the room. And the mother goes out to be with him.

*In the video, Johnny leaves the room, and Peter Levine talks to Susie about what had happened. Susie explains, "I got to push the button that made the siren go." Levine asks, "How did that feel?" and Susie replies, "Feel good! And if I fell in I would still be able to swim, I might get some water in my mouth, but then I would push it out." Peter Levine asks, "So, what did Johnny do?" Susie demonstrates the turning response that Johnny demonstrated earlier. Susie says, "I thought he was already dead," and Levine replies, "Oh no, you must have felt terrible." Susie says, "Yeah, but then mummy jumped in, and they said, oh, he's going to be OK." Now Susie goes back to talking about the toy she got afterwards and the time when she realised that Johnny was going to be OK, and that he had not died. Peter Levine says, "Oh, I bet you were relieved then, I bet you were like . . . [draws a deep breath]" Susie echoes the response and says, "Oh, thank god!" Peter Levine echoes her statements: "Yeah, thank god, thank god, he's OK, he's going to be OK. And you did the right thing, because you went and called mum right away." Susie, "Yes and I saw her get a booboo in her knee."*

Here we see how that narrative part is really taking her through the whole experience. Obviously, this is a different capacity that is not exhibited nearly to that degree with a two-year-old.

*In the video, Susie says, "And everyone was saying he's going to be OK." Peter Levine echoes her statement and emotion: "Yeah, thank god. Can you remember everyone saying that?" Now, Susie is distracted by Pouncer.*

Susie doesn't want to face that image right now. And that's fine. But I kind of gently bring her back.

*In the video, Peter Levine says, "And when you got to the hospital, did you go into the room at the hospital?" and Susie replies, "Yeah, but one room I wasn't allowed to go in . . . but then I could go in." Peter Levine replies, "And then you saw he was OK . . ."*

That was probably the emergency room. Again, this is about reinforcing those moments, those after-moments, the "I have survived" moments.

*In the video, Peter Levine says, "And you said, oh I'm glad you're my brother," and Susie replies, "Yes, but he's still a pain in the neck."*

So you know that she's fine! The trauma's gone for her! Pouncer's relaxed also.

*In the video, Peter Levine and Susie mimic the sound of sirens. Johnny comes in and does the falling game again, now running and jumping, pretending to blow water out.*

Again, we see more exuberance; it's as if his movements are saying, "Hey, I'm alive!"

*In the video, Susie and Johnny are playing, falling off the sofa in all manner of ways.*

You really see their exuberance here. And again, it's very relaxed now. It's relaxed and more active. It's both quieter and exuberant. I want to continue this until I get a particular response that I always look for in connection with drowning, and that's coughing. The shutdown system constricts the smooth muscles in the bronchials, and if the constriction does not go away, the child could easily become more susceptible to bronchial infections and so forth and even asthma. So I want to keep going until we get this response . . .

*In the video, Johnny coughs, and Peter Levine says, "Yeah, cough that water out!" and now Susie is coughing, too. Levine explains the significance of the coughing to the mother, and she explains that Susie watched him cough up a lot of water. Now the teddy bear is included in the playful re-enactment of the incident. Peter Levine has the bear perform a slow-motion fall from the sofa, while Susie yells, "It's OK, bear!"*

"It's OK, bear. It's OK. It's going to be OK." I think Johnny is in graduate school now . . .

## Summary

Both the therapy processes that are outlined in this chapter deal with post-trauma reactions after life-threatening events. The children lived in good families and were securely attached to their parents, but they had severe symptoms and after-effects, because the autonomic nervous system was unable to find its way from a parasympathetic shut-down and freeze response to the healthy defensive responses, coping and joy-filled expression. However, with Peter Levine's specialised and insightful support for autonomic self-regulation, the children were able to find their way from the parasympathetic shut-down, somatisation, and "freeze" response and into healthy defensive responses, coping and joy-filled activities. With this support, the children underwent an almost miraculous development and were able to establish healthy arousal regulation, adaptive self-protection responses, and a sense of trust and confidence in the world.

Severely dysregulated children do not have a secure attachment, and although it is equally crucial to address autonomic regulation in these children, the arousal waves must be embedded in emotionally supportive play that allows the limbic attachment aspect to mature and regulate the autonomic system.

# CHAPTER FOUR

# The limbic compass and Theraplay

"Therapy without risk-taking probably isn't therapy"

(Jukka Mäkelä)

I n this chapter, we first describe the limbic level of mentalization
and the compass for the limbic emotional level. Then we turn to
the Finnish child psychiatrist Jukka Mäkelä's description of
theraplay, and, finally, we review the therapy excerpt that Jukka
Mäkelä presented at the conference.

## The limbic system

The limbic system is functionally associated with emotions and
memory, and, indeed, the system is often called the emotional brain.
It does not have very strictly defined boundaries, and while some
parts of the limbic system act as a general control system for the autonomic nervous system, the brainstem and the neural structures that
are closely associated with the regulation of brainstem structures,
including the hypothalamus, other parts are more closely associated

with the cortex. The limbic system forms the basis for our emotions, connects to the neocortex, and is involved in perceptual and cognitive processes.

The limbic structures are believed to have developed as mammals became more closely attached to their offspring, and the offspring, in turn, responded with attachment behaviour when they were separated from their parents. The limbic system is an emotionally motivating structure that filters internal and external events. The limbic system helps to intensify or dampen arousal and gives perceptions an affective or emotional charge. The area consists of a large number of circuits: thus, emotions are not limited to one emotional circuit, and neither do they have one single centre in the brain (Damasio, 1999). Until the prefrontal lobes are fully developed, the limbic system has a significant influence on the child's behaviour. In regressive behaviour in both children and adults, the limbic system often takes control, overruling rational thinking and acting out immediate impulses, for example, seeking instant gratification or displaying uninhibited expressions of rage (Cicchetti & Tucker, 1994; Lewis, Amini, & Lannon, 2001; Schore, 2003a; van der Kolk, 2000; van der Kolk & McFarlane, 1996).

The limbic system enables the development and refinement of social interactions and, thus, also social emotions such as playfulness, excitement, or sadness. Humans develop the so-called categorical emotions, which are reflected in facial expressions. The categorical emotions are universal emotions, although there is some disagreement about which emotions qualify as universal. Darwin and others mention seven specific categories: joy, sadness/distress, fear, disgust, hatred, surprise, and interest. These emotional states give rise to action impulses, and the limbic system is, therefore, sometimes referred to as the motivation system. In humans, the limbic system enables proto-conversation and arousal regulation by means of emotional intersubjective attunement, which is a precursor of both representation formation and the comprehension of symbols.

## The limbic level of organisation

The emotional limbic level of organisation ranges from around the age of 2–3 months until around the age of 9–12 months. From around the age of 2–3 months, the infant relies less on imitation and gradually begins to choose actions in response to communication. This "conversation", which unfolds in the form of mimicry, gestures, and sounds, is called proto-conversation. Interactions at this age level are non-verbal, and the infant's capacity for preferring stimuli that are not imitative but, instead, constitute proto-conversation supports the development of a capacity to understand others' behaviour as different from the child's own and to internalise others' experience as separate from one's own. Proto-conversations develop and are regulated in the same way as adult conversations (Beebe & Lachmann, 2002; Stern, 1977). The capacity for proto-conversation and arousal regulation through emotional intersubjective attunement is a precursor of both representation formation and the comprehension of symbols. During the first six months of life or so, a normally developing child will develop a natural balance between imitative contact initiatives and proto-conversations that promote the sense of togetherness. Since protoconversations are defined by expressive polarity, such as chaser–chased, they may shift this balance, so that the person's contact is characterised either by fusion and a lack of boundaries or, at the other opposite, by excessive boundaries and conflict-seeking behaviour.

Peter Fonagy (Hart, 2009) suggests that in the infant's earliest consciousness and mental state, he or she does not distinguish between interior and exterior, and that the first developmental project is about achieving a growing sense of distinction. With inspiration from Winnicott's (1967) theory that when the infant looks at the mother's face while she is looking at the infant, the infant actually sees him/herself, Fonagy argues that recurring experiences with affect-regulating mirroring helps the infant understand that emotions do not necessarily spill over into the outside world, and that mental states are different from the physical world. This understanding develops through affect mirroring and attuned responses from the carer, where the infant gradually develops an understanding of his or her inner states and also comes to understand others as psychological beings. There is a difference between the carer's realistic/unmarked emotional expressions and his or her marked expressions. The mirroring unmarked affect expression lets the child know that the carer shares the child's feeling, which implies that the child's affect expression is contagious, while the marked affect expression shows the child that the carer feels *with* the child, but does not feel the same *as* the child.

The marked expression shows the child that the carer is able to contain the child's feeling without being infected or overwhelmed by it. Thus, it is likely that the infant experiences the carer's emotional expression in two different forms: an unmarked and a marked form. The behavioural responses that are associated with unmarked emotional expressions, such as the sight of the mother when she is angry, will be qualitatively different from the responses that occur in connection with a similar marked expression, such as the sight of the mother mirroring the infant's anger. If the carer responds to the child's negative affective expression with an identical emotional expression, the emotion is reproduced in an unmarked, realistic form. The child will be frightened, and the perception loses its symbolic potential. This is equivalent to the clinical description of projective identification as a pathological defence mechanism—which involves projecting undesirable psychological material on to a significant other, with whom the individual then identifies. In the case of projective identification, it can be difficult to sort out who is the sender and who is the recipient of emotions.

Around the age of 6–8 months, we see the emergence of an attachment pattern and attachment behaviour, and the child begins to display anxiety towards strangers. The relationship with the carer becomes a part of the child's internal organisation that is not easily replaced, and others cannot easily take the carer's place and give the child the stimulation he or she needs. The carer becomes a sort of base that the child will return to when tired or insecure. Around the age of nine months, the child is able to build internal representations and to imagine the carer when she is absent. The nine-month-old child is able to recall interactions with others, has internalised the parental representation and has come to expect certain kinds of behaviour (Aitken & Trevarthen, 1997). When the child has formed internal representations of generalised interactions this leads to the attachment patterns that the child is going to rely on in subsequent interactions with others.

Around the age of six to nine months, the child develops the capacity for joint attention with his or her carers, sharing a focus on something other than the dyadic contact. This capacity does not develop until the child is able to attune emotionally with the carer's emotions, not just her actions, and to attain psychological intimacy as well as physical intimacy. The child no longer responds to what the carer does, but gradually becomes much more aware of her mental state. In the dyad, the carer influences the infant's mood modification, that is, how the child should feel, how intensely, and whether he or she should have feelings about particular objects in the environment (Schore, 2003a; Stern, 1977, 2004). The child begins to be able to assign intentions and motivations to others and develops a sense of whether he or she is attuned with others' emotional states. The child not only experiences a rich inner life, with feelings, motivations, and intentions, but comes to understand that others, too, have an inner life. Internal experiences can be shared with others, and the child learns to share attention, intentions, and affective states. Based on early affective attunement experiences, the child discovers the possibility of establishing a field of resonance with the carer. The child learns when an experience can be shared with the carer, and when it remains isolated (Stern, 1985). At this level of maturation, it is, therefore, crucial that the carer or the therapist can bring his or her own feelings into the interaction through engaged, marked mirroring to enable the child to explore his or her experiences of another person's varying mental states.

## The limbic compass

The point of the limbic compass is that our emotional interaction experiences build deep-rooted and non-verbal interaction expectations, which are transmitted from one person to another through mimicry and body language. The flexibility of one's emotional valence and centre of orientation are key elements in limbic–emotional self-regulation and in one's sense of being both securely attached and differentiated from others. This, then, defines the two axes in the compass model for the limbic system (Figure 6). One axis represents the range of positive and negative emotional experiences or valence, while the other axis represents centrism, that is, whether one's focus is on one's own or the other's state and experience. Together, the two axes define four experiential quadrants, which reflect positive or negative emotions associated with either self-experience or the experience of the other. As on the autonomic level, it is important and natural to be able to fluctuate easily among these states and interaction expectations, as that forms the basis of feeling secure, having one's needs met, and perceiving and attuning with others' feelings.

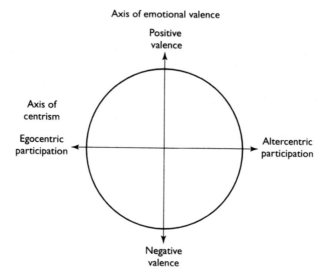

*Figure 6.* The limbic compass.

Thus, the limbic compass is a model of individual interaction expectations and mutual emotional experience of being with others. One axis represents variations in emotional valence, that is, between positive and negative emotional experiences, while the other axis represents variations in centrism, that is, whether the person is focused primarily on his or her own experience or the other's state and experience.

## Limbic interaction quadrants

During the limbic development phase, the child interacts both with carers and other adults and children, and, in these exchanges, the child experiences many different nuances of positive and negative categorical emotions. The child experiences how emotions vary naturally in intensity and how they vary between positive and negative valence. Similarly, the child varies between a healthy, self-centred interest in what he or she finds interesting and satisfying and an interest in others' actions and, later, their internal states. The Norwegian psychologist, Stein Bråten (1993, 1998), has described the child's capacity for altercentric participation. This means that the child has a capacity for engaging in social interaction by first paying attention to the other. In a sense, this means experiencing the other's experience as if one's orientation centre and perspective were centred in the other person. At this time, the child develops the ability to differentiate from others, that is, the ability to combine self-awareness with an awareness of others and to regulate emotionally: that is, a capacity for both ego- and altercentric participation (Figure 7). This capacity develops in part as a result of marked mirroring.

The four experience quadrants produced by these two axes outline emotional expectations in interaction. In the upper left quadrant, we find positive emotions associated with self-centring, such as self-enjoyment or the joy of getting what one wants. Thus, the child has a self-centred focus associated with positive emotions, which leads to a joy-filled expectation of being at the centre of the interaction and having one's needs and desires fulfilled. Related to the upper left quadrant, the child may experience positive emotions associated with attention to others' well-being, such as altruistic desires or the joy of giving someone else something he or she needs. In this case, the child has an altercentric focus associated with positive emotions and is driven by altruistic desires for the other, or positive expectations of

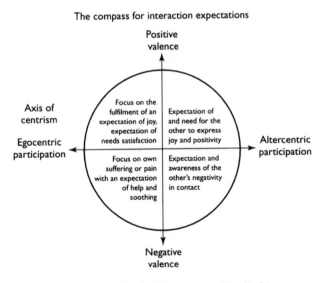

*Figure 7.*   Attunement with the limbic compass. The limbic compass with interaction quadrants (source: Bentzen & Hart, 2013, p. 73).

being able to give the other something of value. An egocentric focus on negative emotions, the lower left quadrant, might involve an appeal for others' attention through symptoms of distress; in that case, the child has a self-centred focus associated with negative emotions, which leads to an expectation of drawing others' attention to his or her own pain or unpleasant internal state. In the last, lower right, quadrant, an altercentric focus on negative emotions is similarly associated with an expectation that others feel anger or envy in relation to oneself.

As on the autonomic level, all these states emerge naturally in interactions, and it is, therefore, also natural to be familiar with them, to experience them from time to time and to be able to shift between them. It is precisely this balanced variability of experiences that allows us to avoid identifying with any single state and, instead, be able to contain them and even to let go of them. Children acquire interaction expectations through attuned interactions with their carers. An older child who has developed the full spectrum of these emotional experiences is able to engage flexibly in all these forms of interactions and to regulate in and out of them.

## Limbic self-protection strategies

On the limbic level, too, the nervous system may be locked into one of these four states as a self-protection strategy, or switch between them in an unbalanced manner. These unregulated states are depicted in the four corner fields in Figure 8. When the child is locked into the limbic compass, he or she may either fluctuate between the extremes on the ego–altercentric axis, or express his or her distress partially through specific emotional discharges, such as anger or anxiety, often through predictable and stereotyped reaction patterns.

In the positive egocentric position, the individual might get stuck in narcissistic self-absorption, where everything is about pursuing one's own needs with no regard for, or sense of, anyone else. All the child's expectations revolve around his or her own satisfaction and outstanding qualities. The positive altercentric experience can lead to self-destructive self-sacrifice, where one is always ready to support others' needs and well-being. In the egocentric negative emotional valence, the individual is trapped in a state of depression or psychosomatic pain, where he or she appeals and desperately seeks help but

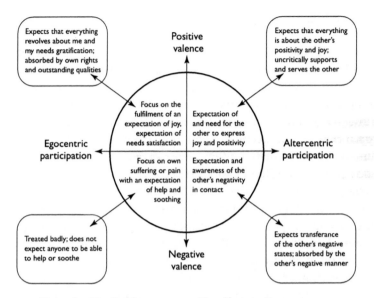

*Figure 8.* The limbic compass with self-protection responses
(source: Bentzen & Hart, 2013, p. 74).

with a sense that others will never provide what he or she needs or show enough consideration. The child perceives it as impossible to get help, or experiences others as unwilling or unable to help. In the alter-centric position, the child might become stuck in an experience of being the object of others' anger, contempt, and sadness, which leads either to an experience of being an innocent victim or to a feeling of being entitled to revenge.

Getting stuck in the limbic compass might involve switching between the extremes of the ego–altercentric axis or take the form of a partial discharge in certain emotional categories: for example, when anger is evoked. Being stuck in this compass means being locked into a role as a bully/torturer, a victim or a helper, or switching between these positions. Switching could involve assigning roles to others where they are either idealised or attributed feelings of hatred or hostility (splitting). It could also involve attributing one's own unbear-able feelings to others (projective identification) or retreating into an internal drama, directing negative feelings at oneself and feeling shame and guilt over other people's actions. These states are often characterised as a borderline disorder. Being stuck on the egocentric pole of the axis can lead to psychopathy disorders.

## Child psychotherapy and balancing the limbic compass

While psychotherapy in relation to the autonomic compass revolved around the pre-verbal dance between the client's and the therapist's basic arousal waves and hedonic moods, interactions in the limbic compass are about pre-verbal attunement, misattunement, repair of attunement, and the establishment of a flexible balance between egocentrism and altercentrism and, thus the development of both the attuned and the security-building sense of attachment and the individuating process of differentiation. This contact requires the therapist to be able to establish affective attunement and a marked mirroring with the client, that is, to be with the client and his or her feelings in both the negative and the positive valence, sensing and containing them without absorbing them, or, as Peter Fonagy puts it, "the capacity to feel with the other but not like the other" (Hart & Schwartz, 2008).

As psychotherapy is about interpersonal learning, it is important to establish attunement processes around both positive and negative emotional valences and to include both egocentric and altercentric impulses and attentional orientations. If the relationship is always focused on the child's problems and negative emotional states, the child might bring this "habit" into relationships outside the therapy room as a new interpersonal contact form, where the exclusively self-centred and problem-focused pattern will hamper the construction of satisfying and equal networks.

The therapist has to enter into the symmetrical human relationship and exchange while maintaining the asymmetrical responsibility, where he or she always considers whether the interaction is helping the child acquire new and healthy emotional and interaction habits. With this model of attunement on the limbic level in mind, we shall now look at Theraplay, a therapy method that has developed tools for expanding and regulating relational limbic attunement.

## Attunement with the limbic compass: presentation of Theraplay by Jukka Mäkelä

As with the autonomic nervous system, there are very few treatment methods that are aimed directly at this level of mentalization. One of the few is Theraplay, which was developed in Chicago during the

1960s and 1970s by the director of Psychological Services of Chicago's Head Start programme, Ann M. Jernberg, together with Phyllis Booth and other colleagues. The Theraplay therapist uses simple and quickly varying interaction games and care-giving situations to create a safe, constantly affirming, and joy-filled interaction that is focused on the present moment and the interpersonal meeting.

In 1967, Jernberg was tasked with identifying children who needed psychological help and referring them to existing services. During the first years of the Head Start programme, she and her team identified almost 300 children who needed help. When they looked for appropriate services in the Chicago area, they realised that it was impossible to find effective treatment options for even a small number of these children. The psychotherapy services available to children were costly and lengthy, and the few existing treatment centres were located far away from the families who needed them. The team realised that they would have to establish a treatment approach that was easy for relatively young mental health practitioners to understand and apply. It seemed obvious to them to base this approach on the playful interaction patterns that come naturally to good enough parents and other adults who like children and enjoying spending time with them.

Jernberg based the new approach on positive interactions between parents and infants. She was inspired by Bowlby, and emphasised having active engagement, eye contact, and direct physical contact between child and therapist. She also emphasised what is going on in the here and now rather than in one's imagination. In her work with emotionally disturbed children, she emphasised the caring relationship between therapist and child, including touch, rocking motions, singing, and physically holding and embracing the child. The team looked for practitioners who had a lively, playful ability to engage children and a strong desire to help them realise their full potential. They found that sad, withdrawn children became livelier, while angry, aggressive children who had been acting out became calmer and more interested in co-operating (Booth & Jernberg, 2009).

Although Theraplay is still used as part of the Head Start programme, it has also spread to other contexts, including early intervention, nurseries and preschools, treatment in the home, foster care and adoption facilities, facilities that promote teaching and care for teenage mothers, residential services, long-term care, etc. (Booth & Jernberg, 2009). The name Theraplay in itself suggests the main difference between this approach and play therapy: in Theraplay, helping the child to be able to engage in interactive, dyadic play is considered a goal in itself. Play is viewed as a therapeutic means, not just a means for conveying internal dramas that need to be understood. The symbolic level is not addressed as a theme—although, of course, many events and episodes have symbolic depths. Instead, play is used as a means of pleasure and joy, mastery and surprise. The rewarding experience of enjoying and finding pleasure by connecting with another person is used to encourage the child to find motivation and confidence in his or her own capacity for engaging in interpersonal attachment. Theraplay seeks to reinforce the basic vitality experience, while play therapy seeks to help children understand themselves and their difficulties better. Theraplay revolves around the child's experiential self-concept, while play therapy revolves around the child's verbal and symbolic self-concept. The use of dyadic, physical, and structured play in Theraplay aims to reinforce the child's capacity for feeling secure and to discover, in this sense of security, elements of him/herself that have not had sufficient room to develop and unfold.

In order to feel secure and develop confidence, the child needs to know that there is a wise and sensitive adult who is looking after him or her. The therapist, therefore, tries to find activities that match the child's actual needs. The therapist guides the session with great sensitivity and is always ready to see and feel the child's initiatives in the interaction. For example, in interactions with children who have difficulties with self-regulation, the therapist makes sure that the play activities do not exceed the children's tolerance thresholds and produce disappointment. The therapist is responsible for creating good experiences in the context of the interaction. Typically, the sessions follow the same basic structure, and the individual activities have a clearly marked beginning and end. More playful activities vary with moments that have a more caring, nurturing character. By providing a clear structure, the therapist sends a clear signal to the child: I will make sure that the world is safe and predictable, and it is safe for you to let go of your need to stay in control (a strategy that probably was useful to you in earlier contexts).

In Theraplay sessions, the therapist challenges the child to take a step towards his or her next level of development—Theraplay aims to stay within the child's zone of proximal development. For one child, that might involve daring to accept close physical contact and nurturing; for another child, it might be to dare to take a more active role in the interaction; for most, it is staying with accepting eye contact. The challenge should be at a level that helps the child succeed. In Theraplay, the goal is to create moments of shared pleasure and success. The therapist invites the child to engage in joint attention and play based on clear and positive instruction and intense positive feedback. The therapist always takes responsibility if an interaction runs off course or misses the mark, both in relation to the child and in relation to the parents. With the dimension of challenge, the therapist says to both the child and the parents, "I want to help you find exciting things that you can do. You have the ability to make good things happen."

Theraplay is a therapy approach aimed at strengthening secure attachment and the capacity for synchronising with others. Developing these capacities gives both the child and the carer increased opportunities for experiencing the psychological benefit of contact and attachment; that is, the emotions that provide direction in our lives and the kind of thinking that makes it easier to make sense of things, thoughts, people, and relationships. Integrating these diverse ways of experiencing the world promotes mental health.

Ideally, Theraplay offers the child optimal challenges, but the therapist is always ready to reduce the challenge if it exceeds the child's capabilities. It is crucial to give the child challenges that are manageable in order to promote feelings of competence, confidence, and agency. In Theraplay, everything should be done in a caring and nurturing way. Close physical contact is an important nurturing element of Theraplay. Since this can be quite challenging, especially for a child who has been neglected and abused, the therapist must always pay close attention in order to sense what the child can handle. Fundamentally, however, close physical contact and touch are never questioned *per se*, as they are crucial aspects of both engagement and nurturing. Everything is done the way an ideal mother or father would do it, and, just as an infant associates mother's milk with nurturing and feelings of being safe, the therapist evokes the child's feelings of pleasure and of being safe and secure by giving the child something sweet to eat and drink, such as chocolate and fruit juice. This nurturing behaviour is not intended to encourage regression but, rather, to answer the questions that went unanswered for far too long during the child's first year of life: "Is anyone assuming full responsibility for looking after me, making sure that my body feels good; good enough to make living worthwhile?"

The four dimensions of Theraplay are:

1.  *Structure*: setting boundaries and ensuring an appropriately structured and secure environment for the child.
2.  *Engagement*: engaging the child in playful interaction while being attuned with the child's states and reactions.
3.  *Nurturing*: meeting the child's needs for soothing, comforting, and care.
4.  *Challenge*: promoting and supporting the child's efforts at succeeding on a developmentally appropriate level.

Jukka Mäkelä describes Theraplay as a psychophysical and intensive parent–child therapy that promotes the child's positive emotional development, helps create a secure attachment pattern, and enhances the parents' sensitivity in relation to their child. The therapy room is designed to contain few distractions and is furnished with soft objects, such as beanbags, a sofa, pillows, etc. It also includes simple things such as soap bubbles, cotton balls, newspapers, skin lotion, feathers, and balloons. The therapist and child sit close together, there is a lot of touching, and the two maintain physical contact. The therapist has the responsibility, and he or she looks at the child with interest and offers eye contact in a non-demanding and meaningful way. The therapist makes positive comments about some of the child's special features, such as the colour of the child's eyes or hair, beauty spots, any special marks or scratches, and positive aspects of the child's appearance; during the activities the therapist also comments on the child's strength, speed, etc.

A typical session lasts about thirty minutes and involves two therapists, as one therapist works with the parents and another works with the child. The sessions consist of simple activities with frequent transitions. The activities consist of interactions of varying intensity, and the beginning and end of each activity are clearly marked. Many of the activities revolve around gearing activation up and then down, relaxing within a field of contact. About one in four sessions is devoted fully to the parents to ensure that they have the necessary support. Initially, the parents observe the child's sessions through a monitor while sitting with their own therapist; after a few sessions, they actively take part in the sessions together with their child.

As Jukka Mäkelä points out, it is important for the child to know that the carer approves of the sessions. The goal is to make room for new emotional experiences without pushing the child into mentalizing, although the therapist often verbalises what he or she notices in the child. The child is allowed to correct the therapist in these observations but does not have to. Theraplay has a clear emphasis on sharing experiences of joy and mastery. The therapist is focused on the here-and-now, on the messages the child sends, and on building attunement processes. The process aims at helping the child to discover him/herself as a person of emotional importance and value in the therapist's eyes. The therapist, therefore, places great emphasis on appreciating the child and showing the child that he or she is special. This is done through micro-regulation processes, as they are the only interaction processes that are open to direct experience.

After this introduction to the maturation of the limbic system and the Theraplay method, we now continue with Jukka Mäkelä's demonstration video of several sequential sessions with the eight-year-old boy, Matias.

## Video clips of Theraplay sessions presented at the conference by Jukka Mäkelä

### Therapy with Matias

Jukka Mäkelä's demonstration video was about the eight-year-old boy, Matias, who had an attachment disorder, and his foster mother. We give the floor to Jukka Mäkelä.

> Matias was an eight-year-old boy, severely abused and neglected in his own family, but, in Finland, it often takes the child protection services many years to figure out whether a child needs placement. Of course, I think that in most cases there should be work going on with the parents in the ways that you're learning about and seeing today, but in this case the parents did not receive any help, and then, after six and a half years, he was taken into custody and placed in a very good foster home. They had had experience with similar children and had managed well. In the clips, you will see the foster mother taking part in the sessions, as the foster father was taking care of the other children at home.

Matias has a lot of problems in school, and the problems mainly come from the fact that he freaks out almost daily. He tries to do his school work, but he fails, and then he is sent away from the classroom: "You're a naughty boy, you go and stand in the corridor; you go to speak to the principal!" And, once a week, the principal has to call his foster mother at home and say, "You have to come and get him, he's freaked out, he's panicking, he's attacking other children", which was very atypical, since he was not normally aggressive, he just had these moments of aggression. At the age of seven he had been diagnosed with ADHD. In Finland, we do not medicate these children first but start with psychosocial interventions. Matias had been given some trial sessions of group therapy with other children in a peer group with other fostered children, where they talk about the stories of their lives, and this freaked him out completely. So he came home in a stupor, and his foster mother had to keep him away from school for some time. He started wetting his bed, soiling himself, and it took many months for him to recuperate from this peer group experience.

So now he came with four other children to this intensive residential Theraplay camp, where the mothers or fathers and the children stay, first for a week and then for another week two or three months later. We have some group sessions as well as separate discussions with the parents, but the main feature is a daily session with the child and the parents from Monday to Thursday (Friday is a group for all children and parents). The clip you're about to see starts from Matias's first day. He had been looking forward to this session, because some of the children in this foster care had been to Theraplay before, and they said to him, "It's a nice place, you get sweets" (which, of course, they do). So Matias came in with very positive expectations. In the morning, when I met him at the breakfast table, he already said that he knew that I would be his therapist, and he was OK with that. But when they were supposed to come, mummy came and said that Matias had freaked out, he was lying on the floor in his room, behind the couch, and she couldn't get him to come. So, we thought that if the mountain will not come to Mohammad, then Mohammad must go to the mountain, so I went to his room, and a few moments later my colleague set up the camera on a shaky chair. This was important. We document everything we do, for many reasons: first, for looking over it with the parents, second, to make sure that everything is all right and safe, and third for supervision, and for other possible purposes.

I lifted Matias up from the floor and said, "I heard that you cannot come to the therapy room. That's OK, I can spend this half an hour with you here, but I don't think that you look comfortable on the floor, so I'll lift you on to the bed."

So I settle him in, and then I say, "You know, I want to see what kind of a boy you are." That's how we always start; clarifying that he has the right to be the child he is, and that I need to get to know him. It's not about me telling him how he should be, but about being interested. I said, "Let's put the pillow here, because the edge of the table would be hard", and then I say, "You've got beautiful golden hair", and then I say, "Oh, I think that you've got all your five fingers there, let's see, one, two, three, four, five. But see, I have a big hand—let's see how much smaller your hand is." I don't remember ever having done it immediately, like this. I mean, when everything is OK, and we have a good rapport, then we do check for different sizes, and I've always thought that when things happen, there usually is a reason. And I thought that what Matias needs most of all right now is to feel safe. Of course, when you go back to Bowlby, how does he describe an attachment figure? Bigger, stronger, wiser, and kind. So, what I think I was doing was making it plain to Matias that I am bigger, I have a bigger hand, and big hands are supposed to be something that encircles the child and takes care of him. And, of course, I am trying to reflect the "kind" quality by making sure that everything is OK, with the pillow there, and using a kind voice. But the wisdom—I don't know!

*In the video, we see Matias sitting on a bed, hiding his face in a pillow. Jukka Mäkelä was also sitting on the bed, close to Matias, with his upper body bending towards Matias. Mäkelä spoke with Matias and sang a sort of lullaby, pausing from time to time to check that Matias was as comfortable as possible by arranging the pillow and then stroking Matias's hair lightly. Matias was almost frozen and seemed very frightened. Mäkelä then held up a finger and invited Matias to count fingers with him. Matias immediately raised his hand to meet Mäkelä's hand, and they counted by touching their fingertips together. First the index fingers, then the middle fingers, etc.*

When he lifted his hand up to meet my hand and to check the size, I thought, "that was a surprise!" I remember the feeling when I said, "Let's check how much smaller your hand is than mine." I thought, "Oh my, this won't work." So I was surprised that he lifted it up, and I thought, OK, we can make this kind of a finger-to-finger contact, because he had already begun to push against my hand. . . . When you do something, the child tends to try to do it himself; that is what mirror neurons are for originally in the ape world. . . . So after that, it was evident that we didn't need to work on basic safety any more. He is feeling safe, otherwise he would not engage in contact with his finger the way he did. So, what happens next in therapy is that we begin to do stuff. Now, I'm not a trauma therapist, so, in another technique, I might be able to begin to work with what was traumatic for him, what made him so afraid and freak out and not be able to come to the therapy room. But I thought that what he needs is experiences of safety, feeling good about himself and feeling capable, so I'm aiming for the pride of mastery, for joy, even though he is so close to being in a terribly traumatic state.

At first, Matias seemed very frightened and vigilant and lacked facial mimicry. Curled up in a freeze response, it seemed that his flight system was about to be activated. Jukka Mäkelä did whatever he could to make the situation as safe as possible. He attempted to lower the arousal level by speaking in a rhythmic, varied voice; he sang a lullaby and used calm movements; and at the same he was insistent and assertive in his attempts at contact. Although Matias had his face in the pillow, he still responded positively to Mäkelä's touch, and Mäkelä was soon able to reduce Matias's unpleasant high-arousal state. In addition, the touch was concealed within a playful activity that only involved the fingertips, so even if Matias's social engagement system had not yet been activated, his arousal level fell sufficiently that the possibility of exchanges on a limbic attunement level seemed possible.

After counting fingers, we always check for wounds. I noticed a tiny scratch that had healed already, but I said anyway, "I'll put some lotion on it." And I was putting lotion on his fingers, and because I think that he is teetering on the edge of falling into traumatic freeze again, I want to make extra sure with him that it feels OK, so I say, "I need to know that this feels OK." Sometimes scratches can smart when you put lotion on them, so I wanted to make sure and asked him to tell me whether it feels OK, and he says, "No, it doesn't smart." So now we have verbal contact also. I repeated that I thought that it might smart, and then I would take it away, because I want to make sure that his fingers feel good. Now, just to support the going-on-being of the therapy, I sing, "I'm lotioning, lotioning, lotioning your fingers, I hope it feels good, I hope it feels nice, that's important for me." Something like that. You can make up the words as you go along.

And then, "yksi, kaksi, kolme, neljä, viisi (one, two, three, four, five)—you might as well learn a little bit of Finnish . . . And now, what I have learnt from my colleague Ilona is that always after counting that there are five, you say, "Just as there should be." You can never be sure that children know how their body should be built.

So, going on to the other hand, lotioning the fingers, then lotioning the hand, and while my hands are slippery I ask him, "Can you draw your hand away?" And he does it, and I say, "Oh, I can't hold your hand. You're so strong!" And then the other hand. The idea here, of course, is that he knows that he *can* get away if he needs to.

*In the video, Jukka Mäkelä now begins a game of "stacking hands", where he and Matias alternately place their hands on top of each other's hands, always moving the hand at the bottom of the "stack" to the top, going higher and higher, building a tower. Mäkelä increased the tempo, speaking in a louder, more excited voice—the game speeds up, until they mess up the rhythm and fall out of step. Matias giggles, but then immediately turns his head away.*

Misattunement! Luckily, Susan told us that misattunements are important. With children who have ADHD, I regularly try to go pretty fast, in a way, in order to tell them that it's OK to be very fast; we need people who are very fast in our society. So we move pretty quickly, and then we slow down, but here I misattuned. I went too fast too soon. He should have had a calm, easy coming down first. He laughed at it, but then you saw the shame reaction, and of course I had to tell him, "You could do it, I just made it too fast. I blundered." And "Let's do it again." I think the answer to shame has to be to correct the attunement. It's not to say, "It's OK", because it's *not* OK to misattune. But doing it again means that we can do it rhythmically in a way that *is* OK.

Matias' anxiety level had now dropped so much that his curiosity was aroused. While Jukka Mäkelä put lotion on his arms, it seemed as if his flight response might have been activated, but when the interaction turned into a game where Matias pulled his arm back, and Mäkelä in turn acknowledged his action by commenting on how strong he was, he moved one step closer to activating the social engagement system and moving into the zone of the limbic compass. Matias grew bolder. His face was now completely free of the pillow, and occasionally he had eye contact with Mäkelä. When the mis-attunement occurred in the fast-paced hand game, Matias seemed to forget about his anxiety for a moment, and his facial mimicry was activated. Then he appeared to be startled because he had been drawn into the field of contact, and he quickly turned his face away. Mäkelä continued talking, as if nothing had happened, and from this moment on, Matias seemed to be in the pleasant part of the autonomic nervous system, and Mäkelä was now able to vary between high- and low-arousal activities within an optimal level. Now, he could continue to work on attunement processes within the limbic compass.

*In the video, they are playing "stacking hands" again. Jukka Mäkelä says, "You were so fast that I couldn't keep up!" Then they move on to a different version, using fist over fist. Mäkelä says, "Boom!" when a fist lands on the fist below. Then he asks Matias, "Can you take them down? This feels really good!"*

When I use fists, that is also to show them that aggression is OK, and that's why I usually say "Boom!" and the child usually begins to say "Boom!" with me, but he didn't, so I toned it down. But now, we had started with his fist at the bottom of the "tower", and I always think that it's important to have a full experience, so if he starts by being at the bottom, the game should also end with his fist at the bottom, and now I noticed that I had misattuned again. So I said, "You know what, we started with you being at the bottom, so let's just see if you can still push it underneath." There's the mattress there, underneath my hand. And I think this is about the first eye contact we had, when he said, "Yes, we started with mine", and then I said, "We'll have to see if you can still stick it under my fist."

*In the video, we see Matias managing to do this, and Jukka Mäkelä makes a sound with his voice—"wroommm!" In a couple of brief exchanges, he first gives Matias some sweets, and then he gently massages his forehead while he speaks to him in a soft, encouraging voice.*

Because he had succeeded, I give him a gold medal; a Pringles is a nice gold medal, and when he takes it then I can admire his teeth, and I say, "You've been given wonderful set of pearly white teeth!" He clearly could not really take this amount of good personal feedback, so he started getting really furrow-browed, so I began to massage his forehead. "All kinds of worries there can be, but no problem. Here, we don't have to think about them."

*In the video, Jukka Mäkelä goes on to massage Matias' feet.*

Now I say, "The sun is so strong, I can't really see the colour of your eyes, so I'll have to turn you sideways." Now, after I've checked his eyes, he's more relaxed on the pillow, and I can begin to work on his feet. Boys are sometimes a bit sensitive about their feet. This mother had taken very good care, and they were clean and nice. With bigger boys, I usually tend to have a wet warm towel, just to make sure that he doesn't have to be self-conscious, I can wash them . . . So I'm commenting, "You have five toes, and you know, the skin is really well taken care of, so I'll just put on some extra lotion." So, if there are wounds you put on lotion, and if there are no wounds you put on lotion, but there's always a rationale to give the child this strong sensation of a massage. I say to Matias that this foot is really good, and he says, "The other foot is not!" And maybe you can't really see his expression, but he's smirking, like, "What are you going to do about that!" And I say, "OK, we'll get to that other foot soon." This toe nail is slightly ingrown, so I massage the cuticle out, and again I make sure that it feels OK for him.

As Jukka Mäkelä moved slightly away from Matias, and the attention turned to a shared third object, Matias' toes, Matias visibly relaxed. His face is relaxed, and he began to engage in conversation and to challenge Mäkelä with a friendly and slightly cheeky smile. Matias now seemed to feel secure enough to explore Mäkelä in a playful way by taking the initiative to challenge him. In this sequence, we see how Matias challenged the balance of ego-altercentric participation ("I know that you might think the other foot is fine too, but I'm still going to challenge your position, which is not the same as mine!") This challenge had a positive emotional valence and occurred in an atmosphere where Matias' self-esteem seemed to have grown.

I so enjoyed the pushing away, and it's something that all children do. If they don't do it naturally, then we tell them to push us away, as a game. In a way, it's just to show their strength and their capability, but it also gives them this idea that "I can push you away if I need to."

*In the video, Jukka Mäkelä has taken Matias's feet in his hands and asked Matias to push him over with his feet. Mäkelä offers just enough resistance to still allow Matias to knock him over. Next, Matias and Jukka Mäkelä begin to blow a cotton ball back and forth between them. Matias' face is open and alive now, and he laughs several times. Next, they do pat-a-cake, varying the pace.*

This is just a cotton ball and a piece of paper; we call it cotton ball football. We blow it towards each other, and the idea is that if he can get it to topple over the edge of the paper on my side, he gets a point, and if I can do it on his side, then I get a point. And with children it's very important to first make sure that they get several points. It's a fun activity, because when you both blow, the cotton ball jumps high into the air, and then I can comment on it: "Wow, I've never seen it jump so high!" Which is true *in the moment*. The authenticity comes from this moment, not from the generalisations.

*In the video, Matias now sits on a pillow in Jukka Mäkelä's lap. Taking Matias's hand in his, Mäkelä takes Matias's finger and first pushes his own nose while making a deep "honk!" sound and then Matias's nose next while making a high-pitched "beep" sound.*

That was the end of the first session: the calming down, the relaxation, which of course is very unnatural for him at his age. So, again, it's just having this, in a way, freakish, not-real relationship with some crazy guy who's doing all sorts of funny stuff and giving him sensations and experiences that he wouldn't get otherwise. Because I am a male, I always have a pillow on my lap and put the child on the pillow, to offer the security of distance. But in fact he was exceptionally good for his age at snuggling in from the first moment. Just asking a child to relax would not work. But playing something, like "Beep! Honk!" usually really distracts the child from not being able to relax and gives him or her the possibility of feeling something of the relaxation.

Matias was half an hour early for the next session, waiting at the door to the therapy room. I did not ask any questions afterward, about whether it would be all right for him to come, and I never asked him what he felt when he couldn't come, because Theraplay is a form of therapy where we work on new experiences. It's not about working through bad experiences, except for a few situations: when a child has been seriously physically traumatised or sexually abused, we tend also to speak about what these new experiences are needed for. That "I know you have been touched in ways that have hurt you; I know that you have been touched in ways that adults should not touch children. So here I'm demonstrating to you what it feels like to be touched in another way. In a way in which adults should touch children, taking care, nurturing, having fun." And I say this even to very young children, if there is knowledge of abuse, especially sexual abuse. Bigger children might say things like, you know, "Don't touch me, you faggot", and then I say, "Oh, OK, I see that you know what it is when adults touch you in bad ways, so I want to tell you that *this* is taking care of children. *This* is what adults should do with young people. You know what they *shouldn't* do", trying to help them to distinguish between these two ways of touching.

I've only included a few crucial things from the next sessions.

*In the video, we now see a new room where Matias is sitting in a large beanbag chair in the corner. Matias playfully pushes Jukka Mäkelä, who falls backwards in an exaggerated tumble, kicking his feet in the air. Mäkelä says to Matias, "That was really strong, I flew half-way across the room!"*

As everyone knows who has played with small children, it's so much fun for an adult to put some extra effort into exaggerating stuff that happens. And I was never taught this in therapy training before I learnt Theraplay: that we can give something strong from ourselves. Instead of simply picking up from what the child does, we can make these exaggerations.

*In the next clip, Jukka Mäkelä and Matias play with soap bubbles. Mäkelä blows bubbles, and Matias pops them. At one point, Matias stubs his finger against the wall, and Jukka Mäkelä immediately takes the finger and blows on it.*

I'm challenging him to see how many soap bubbles he can pop before they drift down to the floor. With another child, I might just pick one soap bubble and make them really concentrate on that one. But, as I mentioned before, with children who have ADHD I tend to get them really revved up and then let them calm down. Simply asking children to calm down does not help them regulate.

Here he hits or touches his hand against the wall, which offers the adult an opportunity to offer nurturing. I exaggerate the incident by blowing on his finger and making sure that his hand is OK, even though, of course, it didn't really hurt. The idea is to notice anything that happens and tend to it as if it were a major thing, to tell the child that it is our responsibility as adults to take care of children.

*In the video, we now see two games, first thumb wrestling, where Jukka Mäkelä supports Matias's hand and arm and lets him win. Next, they arm wrestle standing up, and again, Mäkelä lets Matias win, tumbling over with exaggeration, feet in the air.*

In Finnish, we call this kind of arm wrestling "sailor's wrestling"; it's a good way to show the child his or her strength. And thumb wrestling is excellent too, because even quite young children are actually are so good, so quick, that it's very difficult to beat them, and that lets them take pride in their mastery.

Training in the limbic compass is about attunement, misattunement, and especially the repair of misattunement processes through marked mirroring, where the person who is higher in the asymmetrical hierarchy is responsible for giving the child experiences that will promote the development of the child's interaction capacity and positive self-esteem. This process is initiated in a zone of positive emotional valence, which supports the child's development of self-esteem; an important part of the limbic process. In many of the activities and games that Jukka Mäkelä used with Matias, Mäkelä gave himself a handicap and allowed Matias to win. This type of self-imposed handicaps occurs in almost all mammals when adult animals play with young animals. Only when the child's zone of proximal development (regardless of biological age) has reached the socialisation stage does the child have to learn to handle losing.

*In the video, we now see a classic trust exercise. Matias is standing, leaning his back lightly against Jukka Mäkelä's hand and keeping his body erect, while Jukka gently pushes him from side to side. Initially, Matias is slightly insecure and seeks eye contact with Mäkelä, who confirms with his eyes that everything is all right. Then Matias allows his head to sway gently with the movement, laughing. He allows himself to be pushed gently forwards and backwards, while Mäkelä gradually increases the arc. Meanwhile, Mäkelä makes supportive sound effects with his voice—a descending wooo-mmm sound every time Matias lets himself glide into the short fall and is caught.*

This is what I call a trust pendulum. The idea is that the child stands, and I start to make him or her swing back and forth. At first, I keep my hands very close together, and then I gradually make the arc wider. I was very surprised that Matias was so good at it, because often children are more unco-ordinated. Immediately, when I noticed that he is good at it, it was easy to demonstrate to him how capable he is. And he is not so sure yet, as you can see from his expression. "Can I do this sideways too?"

*In the video, Jukka Mäkelä and Matias are now engaged in a sword fight with foam rubber "swords". Both Matias and Jukka Mäkelä were clearly engaged and excited; they are laughing, out of breath, and fully using their bodies. Mäkelä says, "Keep coming, keep coming, keep coming!" Suddenly, Mäkelä says, "Stop!" and Matias stops immediately with a look of pride on his face.*

These swords are used for insulating water pipes. They are really cheap in the hardware store, and they are so thin that even young children can hold them in their hand. When we do the fencing, I always tell them to go on as hard as they can and as fast as they can, and when I say stop, they have to freeze! The idea is to get them excited and then to show them the strength that they have in themselves to freeze. I have yet to meet a kid who doesn't get that immediate freeze thing, and then we start again and go on. I think that demonstrates that there are many ways of being strong; that being strong is being able to take control of your movements.

By now, Jukka Mäkelä and Matias were so attuned, and misattunements were repaired so quickly, that Mäkelä could begin to challenge the boy's prefrontal system and its impulse inhibition capacity. Mäkelä had included it in previous activities: for example, by asking Matias to wait for a "Go!" signal before pushing away with his feet to knock Mäkelä over. Gradually, Mäkelä raised the bar: When he called "Stop!" Matias had to stop instantly. Matias had previously had trouble stopping: for example, when a teacher asked him to, which had caused impulse breakthroughs and serious altercations between him and his teacher. By introducing the impulse inhibition at times when Matias had a capacity for impulse inhibition and was able to stop, Mäkelä managed to offer the opposite experience, acknowledging Matias for the resource he displayed in this ability to stop, and enabling Matias to feel pride and joy in his mastery.

*In the video, Matias is lying in Jukka Mäkelä's lap while Matias's foster mother is looking for a sweet that is hidden under Matias's shirt. Matias laughs several times and makes eye contact with Mäkelä and his foster mother. When the mother finds the sweet, she pops it into Matias's mouth, and he accepts it easily.*

So this is when the mother comes in. As I said, parents can come in either very early or right at the end. This mother wanted to come only for the last two sessions, and she was afraid that there would not be time enough. The first time she came, she joined my activities, and the second time she was in charge of the session and I supported her. First, she looked for sweets; I had hidden little goodies on Matias. For many parents it's not easy to touch in a safe way, which means touching without being too surprising, not in a way that tickles. Matias's mother had practised with Ilona, my colleague, who was working with the mother while they observed Matias's sessions through a montior. So now she knows how to touch in a way that is OK for Matias. She was surprised by how well it went, because, she said, Matias never accepted anything from her. That was one of her worries: that this just wouldn't work, because it had never worked before. But because it was part of the game, it was possible for Matias to forget that this wasn't supposed to happen.

*In the next clip, the foster mother, Jukka Mäkelä, and Matias are playing with soap bubbles, and Matias tries to pop them as fast as he can. Matias says, "I can do this even with my toes!" Mäkelä stops what is going on to ask, "Is it possible?! I have never seen anybody do it just with their toes!" Matias then popped the bubbles with his toes, looking immensely proud of his achievement and his foster mother voiced her admiration.*

Now comes the last session, where I'm just supporting mummy. She has planned this session and practised the activities with Ilona, and now she's doing it with Matias. When popping soap bubbles with his fingers, Matias offered us another surprise—children are so inventive. She had asked him to pop them with thumb, forefinger, middle finger, index finger, and little finger, but then he started going back, doing it in reverse, and she noticed that and commented on how good and capable he is, so I could say, "You are so good at noticing what Matias does."

*In the video, the foster mother and Matias are now playing with foam rubber bats and balloons. They use the bat to hit the balloon, passing it back and forth as in a badminton match, and there is lots of laughter. Next, the*

*foster mother holds a sheet of newspaper stretched taut between her hands,*
*and Matias breaks it with a karate chop, striking it as hard as he can.*

We had asked her to plan activities she could do at home. Activities
that Matias had enjoyed, and which she could imagine building into
their relationship. She was the one to suggest balloon volleyball and
then karate chopping newspapers. In newspaper karate, the idea is
that the parent takes hold of smaller and smaller and smaller pieces of
paper as fast as she can, and the child has to chop them up—without
hitting the parent. This, again, is one of these elements of sharing joy,
of sharing pride.

*In the next part of the video, the foster mother is holding Matias in her*
*arms. He is leaning against a pillow and looks up into her eyes from time to*
*time. He is drinking from a carton of apple juice. Matias and his mother are*
*in intense contact, and she supports him as he drinks. At one point, he signals*
*that he needs a little break, and she notices this signal as well as the subse-*
*quent signal that he was ready to begin drinking again.*

In this sequence, Matias almost resembles a baby drinking from a
bottle, as he activates his sucking reflex and his snuggle response in
the foster mother's arms. He seems to be reclaiming "lost ground". At
the same time, he is challenged on this age level by being asked to
drink the apple juice as fast as he can. This activates the autonomic
nervous system in terms of activating the reflexes and the secure base
that enables the development of the limbic system while also engaging the eight-year-old boy's need for competitive games, a feature of
the prefrontal system.

She was by nature not a very cuddly mother, not with her other children either; but she was very physically active, she was into cross-
country skiing and stuff. So I wasn't at all surprised that she thought
that these very strong activities would be the best for her and Matias.
And it turned out that they took up skiing also and went on long
skiing trips. But the biggest surprise was that the very next day when
they went home, and Matias went back to school, no one phoned from
school, and Matias came back and started tell her about everything
that had happened during the school day. That was a total change,
because previously he had come home and disappeared into his own
room and would not be in contact with the rest of the family. In fact,
it has been a few years since this happened, and it has continued, and

Matias is doing very well at school. There was no need for medication or any other ADHD treatment, and the neurologist was a bit astounded that Matias was doing so much better. I don't know if there was any ADHD at all; I think that these were just the almost panicky situations in which he could not control himself. And the fact that he found this way to contact with a mother whose strength was in physical prowess was important for him.

## Summary

Matias had grown up against a background of severe neglect. The therapy process outlined in this chapter was characterised by a focus on attachment by means of attunement processes, which are mediated by the limbic system.

The point of the Theraplay process, thus, was to work with Matias' arousal and affect regulation capacity through dyadic interactions in an asymmetrical relationship that aimed to strengthen his social capacity and enable him to practise with peers at a later stage. With Jukka Mäkelä as a safe "caravan leader", the therapy process established a secure base by means of up- and down-regulated play where Matias was able to rehearse his interaction capacity through carefully matched micro-regulation processes. When misattunements occurred, they were quickly repaired. Jukka Mäkelä's film clip was in Finnish, so probably no one in the audience understood a single word of it, but all the core elements of the therapy could still be easily seen and understood.

As mentioned in the previous chapter, therapy with severely dysregulated children who do not have secure attachment must address autonomic regulation and embed the arousal waves in emotionally supportive play so that the limbic attachment aspect can promote the development and regulation of the autonomic system.

# CHAPTER FIVE

# The prefrontal compass and developmentally supportive conversations with children

"Love is not enough. There has to be some substance also that the child can use to develop. There has to be room for agency, where the adult provides time, physical and mental space and recognition of the child as a self-organising agency. There has to be room for and acceptance of the child's responses"

(Haldor Øvreeide)

The frontal lobes are the top tier of the triune brain. In humans, the frontal lobes make up about a third of the neocortex. The area, which includes the prefrontal cortex, emerged around the old limbic system and is the brain's most complex area. Among other functions, it enables abstract thinking. It connects to all the reaction paths in the brain and converts signals from all sensory areas into images, thoughts, and bodily states that are represented continuously. The prefrontal cortex is crucial for maintaining emotional stability. In the previous chapter, we discussed the limbic level of mentalization and the limbic compass and described Theraplay as a method aimed at the limbic level of organisation. In this chapter, we focus on the mentalizing level of organisation and the prefrontal compass, that is, the neural structures and stages of maturation associated with this level. We also present the Norwegian psychologist Haldor Øvreeide's description of the dialogue-based method of developmentally supporting conversations with children, which targets this level of organisation. In closing, we describe the demonstration video that Haldor Øvreeide presented at the conference and comment on some of his reflections based on the three compass models.

## The prefrontal cortex

The prefrontal cortex forms impulses and plans for action sequences and is especially highly developed in primates, in particular in humans. In humans, the prefrontal cortex is approximately twice as big as it is in other primates. It co-operates with the body-sensing areas in the parietal lobes, and together they constitute much of what is typically defined as intelligence today. The prefrontal cortex plays an important role in recalling stored memories such as facts, rules, etc., and as a working memory, which provides a huge degree of flexibility. Alexander Luria called the prefrontal cortex the "organ of civilisation" (Goldberg, 2001).

The area is a source of mental flexibility because it is capable of altering thoughts and actions based on altered associations. It controls primitive behaviour and basic emotions by inhibiting impulses and taking over control from the reflexive instinctive systems and from the emotional limbic structures. The multiple connections between the prefrontal cortex and the rest of the neocortex are the source of human imagination and the ability to form complex ideas based on a multi-modal sensory system. The social maturation of the prefrontal cortex develops the human mentalization function, which includes the capacity for self-reflection and an inherent ability to decode what is going on in another person's mind. It is the prefrontal cortex that enables us to make sense of perceptions, predict the future, and select certain thoughts, emotions, and sensations for further consideration while choosing to ignore others, deeming them less significant. The prefrontal cortex lets us go on mental journeys that are also related to the future. It lets us recall situations from our past, imagine the future, and integrate our past, present, and future. It enables special subjective experiences. It is this area that makes mankind so unique. Our ability to make choices is guided by prefrontal calculations, which include an assessment of the current situation compared with our desires, values, and assumptions about the consequences of a given action. Much of the prefrontal area is uniquely human and enables us to make choices in situations that are not about finding a specific, objectively correct solution.

The prefrontal cortex is the area where emotional and mental impressions are put together and given direction, and actions are planned, where mental images can be held and manipulated, and where plans and visions are formed. This area lets us pick one strategy over another, enabling us to suppress or manage emotions or act differently in order to handle a situation better.

The orbitofrontal cortex, which is situated close to the limbic system and which represents the top of a hierarchy where the lower levels are the limbic system and the autonomic nervous system, represents the apex of emotional regulation. The connections between the orbitofrontal cortex and the amygdala mediate the modulation of behaviour by means of reward and punishment, and the orbitofrontal cortex is involved in the joy-filled qualities of social interactions. The orbitofrontal cortex makes sense of behavioural and unconscious reactions that have already been initiated by limbic structures, and it handles impulse inhibition, that is, our ability to inhibit the activation of maladaptive actions. Fully developed orbitofrontal functions enable the organism to balance internal needs and external realities, and the structure plays an important role in affect regulation, impulse control, and reality testing.

The cingulate gyrus and the orbitofrontal cortex are also involved in the formation of object constancy. We need internalised internal representations to attune our behaviour by initiating certain responses and inhibiting others. The presence of this capacity indicates that the child has acquired the capacity for grasping that an object exists permanently in time and space, and that the information can be recalled at a later time when the object is no longer present. The orbitofrontal cortex makes it possible to modulate and contain intense affect and process complex symbolic representations. It enables a child who is experiencing negative feelings to form an internal representation of a comforting other. The orbitofrontal cortex plays a key role in giving rational thinking an emotional dimension and that the mentalization is linked to our feelings. Feelings help us make sense of our thoughts, and they make some things feel more meaningful than others.

## The mentalizing level of organisation

The third level of mental organisation matures from around the age of 8–12 months. Among other functions, it expands a feeling by adding our thoughts about the feeling: what we now refer to as the mentalization capacity. The maturation of this level of mental organisation is highly dependent on stimulation and requires that the carer is able to engage in socialisation of the child, where the child's maladaptive behaviour is inhibited. The inhibitory functions of the prefrontal cortex are internalised through culturally conditioned and socially transmitted behaviours. The neural circuits in the prefrontal cortex have a high degree of plasticity and are influenced by experiences and learning processes, and they take a long time to mature. The frontal lobes are not fully developed until the age of around 20–25 years and are, thus, the latest maturing structure in the human brain (Goleman, 2003).

With the development of the frontal lobes, the child begins to perceive a link between the past, the present, and the future, which is an important condition for distinguishing between interaction and relationship. The child is able to preserve interactions over time and, thus, engage in relationships. It is in this area that we experience feelings of anxiety or regret. Development in this area is huge, and many child therapy methods engage this level of organisation, from role-playing and narrative methods to cognitive, mentalization-based, and systemic therapy forms. At the age of twelve months, the child is able to inhibit certain impulses in order to realise others and to sense different options. At the age of one-and-a-half to two years, the dorsolateral prefrontal cortex matures, enabling the child to develop more complex symbolic representations, which we shall look at in the following chapter in our discussion of the second growth spurt. This symbolisation capacity forms the basis for the development of language. At the age of 12–18 months, the child lives in an egocentric world and is amazed when it becomes clear that others are able to have distinctly different thoughts and feelings. The child does not understand that the mother does not feel what the child feels (Fonagy, 2005). At the age of fourteen months, the child begins to perceive others' pain and tries to help: for example, by calling an adult. Only at the age of 20–24 months does the child attempt to comfort the other or display other forms of nurturing behaviour (Karr-Morse & Wiley, 1997). At this time, the child begins to develop a capacity for empathy, where the child senses his or her own subjective state, which he or she then projects on another person or object.

One-year-old children are able to distinguish between emotional expressions in others, reach conclusions based on this emotional content, and use this information in their considerations about others' behaviour. For example, when the child is uncertain about whether to cross a visual gap to reach the mother, he or she will check the parents' facial mimicry and use this emotional information to modulate his or her own behaviour in a process known as social referencing. Until the age of eighteen months, the child gradually improves his or her ability to co-ordinate his or her own and the carer's mental state in relation to a third object or person. This intentional communication is evident in that the child begins to point, is able to follow the direction of another's gaze and begins to use gestures to indicate an object.

Feelings of shame or embarrassment begin to emerge about the age of 12–14 months, when the child's joy-filled excitement peaks (Schore, 1994, 2003b). The capacity for shame probably evolved as an effective socialisation strategy. When feelings of shame occur, they immediately inhibit the child's curiosity and feelings of pleasure and put an end to explorative behaviour, which is why Schore describes shame as causing the deflation of narcissistic affect. The shame mechanism regulates the child's omnipotent, grandiose, manic, excited high-arousal state and deflates the feeling of omnipotence. Shame is a mechanism that may reduce the child's arousal, which leads to a more balanced self and is, thus, able to drive the developmental process forward. Shame experiences are important for the attainment of self-regulation and the superego structure. The child's shame capacity is vulnerable and has to be attuned in a respectful way to develop adaptively. In child therapy, however, it is essential to remember that prohibition, commands, and sensible talks cannot be used to promote maturation until the preceding autonomic and limbic functions have been integrated and connected with conscious prefrontal control mechanisms.

The ability to distinguish acts that belong in a fantasy realm or a symbolic representation from acts that belong in the real world and

real-life relationships is crucial for the child's personality development. This capacity for discrimination develops in stages between the
age of fifteen months and four years through a co-ordination of experiences that gradually enable the child to associate internal states
with symbols and language and to co-ordinate his or her reality with
another's reality. In psychological terms, this is often referred to as the
capacity for reality correction. At the age of 15–18 months, the child
becomes more aware of the possibility of sharing experiences with
others through linguistic meaning and context. In the rapidly progres-
sing process of language development, the child's attention is drawn
away from the inner world and pulled towards phenomena that can
be described verbally and, thus, shared with others. This may sow the
seed for a profound separation between the non-verbal inner flow of
sensory impressions and experiences on the one hand and the child's
perceived identity and self-concept on the other.

Around the age of eighteen months, the child begins to be able
to use symbols, and begins to develop a capacity for symbolic play,
including "pretend play". During this period, the child is still only
able to engage in parallel play and has a limited capacity for introducing new elements into the play context. Only when the child is
able to grasp that the other person has a different centre, based on his
or her own subjective experiences, does the ability to take on another's
role and engage in role-playing begin to emerge; this does not happen
until around the age of four years (Neisser, 1993; Trevarthen, 1993a,b).
When the zone of proximal development includes the integration of
roles, language, fantasy, and reality, there is a wide range of therapeutic methods that can be used to stage internal partial representations and emotions.

While the ability to maintain sustained internal representations is
established around the age of twelve months, the capacity for forming
mental representations of others' mental representations does not
emerge until around eighteen months. The capacity for forming
mental representations of others' mental representations helps the
child develop self-boundaries, as the child can now distinguish
between his or her own and others' experiences and internal representations. The child begins to develop a sense of how others perceive
him or her and to be able to grasp aspects of another's perspective; this
includes the insight that taking another child's toy will make that child
angry and upset. The capacity for feeling specifically directed anger

and expressing it verbally rather than physically and the development of social self-regulation and self-soothing behaviours are common themes in therapy and key aspects of the child's prefrontal capacity.

## The prefrontal compass

Although the prefrontal cortex begins to mature around the age of 6–9 months, most of the development of the cognitive function and the mentalizing function in the prefrontal cortex takes place after the first wave of maturation, and these skills are, therefore, described in the following chapter. However, simple versions of both prefrontal axes are already in place at this level of maturation, and, therefore, we take a brief look at the final compass model in relation to the triune brain here and revisit it in the next chapter, which deals with the second maturation, or growth spurt.

In the prefrontal compass, the two axes relate to need management and mentalization. Impulses for satisfying one's own needs and desires stem from the limbic and autonomic levels; when they reach the prefrontal level, impulses may either be inhibited or volitionally activated. Mentalization is about the ability to "see oneself from the outside and others from the inside" and to imagine the possible consequences of one's actions: imagining both interpersonal reactions and future consequences of one's urges and desires. A high level of reflective functioning implies mastery of these skills, which means that awareness and reflections on emotions and actions on reflections change and integrate these same emotions and actions. On the other hand, a simplistic or low level of reflective functioning means acting and feeling without knowing why, or being trapped in more primitive, concrete, reality-distorted modes of thinking that have little to do with any external reality (Figure 9).

## Prefrontal interaction quadrants

As in the other compasses, it is a state of balanced flexibility that enables the person to escape identification with the individual states and, instead, be able to contain them and, sometimes, to let go of them.

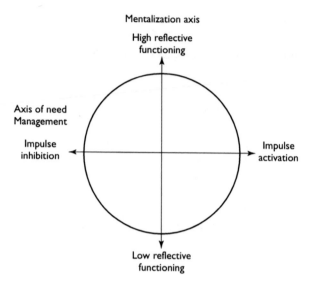

*Figure 9.*   The prefrontal compass.

As on the autonomic and limbic levels, a "healthy" nervous system that has developed a capacity for self-regulation will self-regulate in and out of these states with ease and be able to vary between them. All adults and children who have been socialised carry an internalised moral sense that contains both more and less mature elements. The primitive superego and its commands and prohibitions let the child quickly effect powerful impulse inhibitions and activations, even if the desire and need system wants something else. For example, it is helpful if the primitive prefrontal inhibition can engage immediately to inhibit the child's impulse to act out a burst of anger. Reflection takes time, and before it is concluded the impulse might have long since been acted out. Sometimes, life requires us to be able to effect powerful impulse inhibitions or activations, even if our desires and needs call for something else (Figure 10).

The simplistic reflective function begins to emerge in the second year of life, and even adults with a well-developed mentalization capacity are occasionally overwhelmed by primitive states and feelings and resort to simplistic explanations and perceptions. In both children and adults, it is, therefore, common to find simplistic mentalization, while it is relatively rare to find a stable capacity for reflective mentalization.

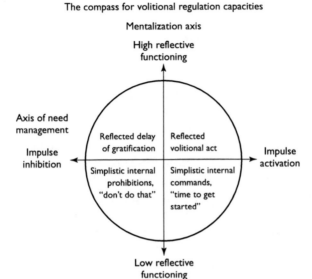

*Figure 10.* Dialogue with the prefrontal compass. The prefrontal compass with interaction quadrants (based on Bentzen & Hart, 2013, p. 84).

When we look at the four experiential quadrants, impulse inhibition with high reflective functioning corresponds to inhibiting an urge or impulse with a view to delaying gratification: for example, by remaining loyal to a close friend even if one is angry with him, because one does not want to hurt him. Through impulse activation based on a high reflective function, the child might, for example, carry out a less attractive task or action in order to obtain a subsequent benefit. Examples include doing one's homework in order to get the good marks required to enrol in a particular study programme or school, or going for a walk when all one wants to do is stay inside and roll down the blinds, because one knows that the fresh air and exercise will help lift the blues.

When the impulse inhibition stems from the low reflective function, the impulse comes from the archaic superego: "No, I mustn't!" Moderate levels of shame help the child regulate his or her relationship with the outside world and serve as a signal for change and self-correction. The child begins to sense when it is best to inhibit one's arousal level and possibly give up a behaviour that is presently gratifying, but which bothers others. When the impulse activation stems from the low reflective capacity it is perceived either as an order from the same archaic superego, "You *must* . . .", or as an attempt to act in way that the parents have defined as morally superior.

### *Prefrontal self-protection strategies*

As in the autonomic and limbic compasses, the four quadrants in the prefrontal compass may become fixated, take on extreme expressions, or cause an unregulated fluttering from one self-protection strategy to the next that might reflect neurotic states in this compass (Figure 11).

In the simplistic, impulse-inhibiting position, the child might have unrealistic visions of disaster or threatening, judgemental internal voices from the superego that threaten dire consequences if the impulse is not inhibited. In the impulse-activated, simplistic position, the child might compulsively fill his or her everyday life with "good deeds" in order to ward off rebuke from the internal judge or the disaster that the child imagines will be unleashed if he or she does not do everything to perfection.

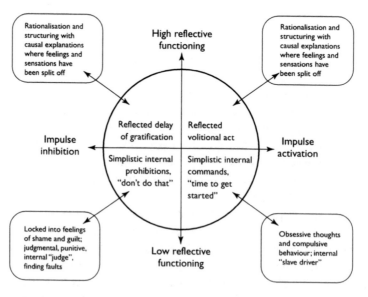

*Figure 11.*   The prefrontal compass with self-protection strategies
(source: Bentzen & Hart, 2013, p. 85).

In the impulse-inhibited highly reflective position, the child might be exhausted by the constant effort to empathise with, understand, and explain his or her own and others' mental states to the degree that pleasurable impulses are always inhibited. In the impulse-activating highly reflective position, there will always be a good reason to do good deeds and to sense the joy this brings, but without sensing one's own needs or boundaries. Thus, the child does not allow him/herself the time to engage in the necessary rest and states of relaxation. Even worse, being locked into the highly reflective position means that the prefrontal rational causal explanations and structuring capacities are split off from emotions, empathy, and sensations of pleasure and discomfort.

## Child psychotherapy and balancing the prefrontal compass

A wide range of therapy and treatment interventions target the rational level of mentalization, from role-playing games and narrative methods to cognitive, mentalization-based, and systemic therapy approaches. At the conference, interventions aimed at this level were beautifully represented by the Norwegian psychologist, Haldor Øvreeide, who presented his approach to structuring and empathic conversations with children, and Eia Asen, who is the director of the Marlborough Family Service in London, who presented the multi-family multi-systemic therapy that the clinic is known for around the world.

While the work in the two previously discussed compasses was preverbal, the psychotherapeutic effort in the prefrontal compass is orientated towards the verbal area and aims to balance impulse-activation and impulse-inhibition while improving the reflective capacity to acknowledge and contain increasing ranges of emotion. In addition, other activities are introduced that give the high reflective capacity a break by inviting calm and relaxed internal states that free the child from the need to be constantly vigilant. The process may include a mix of narrative dialogues and self-observation of bodily sensations, mental images, internal representations, and emotions, as well as reflections on one's own relationship with others. Together, the therapist and the child, and possibly the parents, co-construct new mental images and narratives that are integrated and balanced with structures in both the limbic and the autonomic system. In this process, the goal is to encourage and enable the child and the parents to take ownership of larger and more expanded parts of themselves.

In psychotherapy aimed at the early levels of maturation in the prefrontal cortex, it is important to remember that the connections have to go in both directions: reaching "down" to connect with the limbic emotional states and autonomic arousal processes and maturing "up" to enable a more modulated and reality-based self-perception and perception of the outside world. As the primary development of the prefrontal cortex begins around the age of one year and continues into the early twenties, this maturation process involves multiple stages and levels. In this and the following chapter, we look at two forms of therapy that address the maturation of the prefrontal level and rational mentalization. In the present chapter, we begin with the well-known Norwegian child and family therapist Haldor Øvreeide's developmentally supportive conversations with children.

## Dialogues with the prefrontal compass: a presentation of developmentally supportive conversations with children by Haldor Øvreeide

Haldor Øvreeide works with children and parents, together with his wife and colleague, Reidun Hafstad. Since 1989, they have framed their work within a developmentally supportive perspective. In 1989 in the Netherlands, they met Maria Aarts, who, at that time, was developing what would become the Marte Meo method. One of the focal points of Reidun Hafstad and Haldor Øvreeide's work is the degree to which children's development depends on stable relationships with adults who are able to understand and meet their needs for support and care.

After some years of training and supervision in Marte Meo, Haldor Øvreeide found that when he used what he considered basic principles of developmentally supportive communication in his exchanges with the children, the children actually wanted to stick around, and they wanted to tell him things that it seemed they had never previously articulated or even thought of. They expressed themselves in a more authentic way than he had seen before. The most important discovery, however, was that when the child fell into a better form of communication, the parents seemed to see their child in a completely new light. Suddenly, there was a complete transformation in the parents' way of relating to, and caring for, their child. They began to relate to their child in a way that sprang from real interest and a desire to do something good for the child rather than feelings of "ought to" and "should". Since then, Haldor Øvreeide has always had the parents present during his conversations with children in order to give them an opportunity to see, hear, and experience their child in a new light. Together with Reidun Hafstad, he has developed this approach into a more systematic intervention method with children. Another key factor in developmentally supportive communication, however, is unpredictability. "It's risky," says Haldor Øvreeide, "you never know what will happen, how it will happen and when it will happen. The now moments, they come and go."

The underlying understanding behind developmentally supportive conversations with children is that children's development and quality of life depend on stable relationships with adults who are able to understand and meet their needs for care and support. In a treatment context, the key is to establish a natural, developmentally supportive dialogue that leads to a healthy intersubjectivity between parents and children. The goal of child therapy is to initiate, or reestablish, this intersubjectivity between parents and children, whether the focus of the treatment is developmental support for the adult or a therapeutic process for the child. One way of achieving this goal is through triangulated conversations (Figure 12).

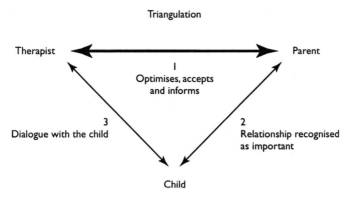

*Figure 12.* Triangulated communication
(source: Haldor Øvreeide's PowerPoint slides from the conference).

When the focus is on the child, the therapist can help the child express his or her needs and capacities. This, in turn, can enable nuanced observations of the child, which can lead to more respectful and caring reactions from the parents. When the focus is on the parents, the therapist's dialogue with the parents can help them clarify and express their sense of responsibility, their caring intentions, and their realistic limitations in relation to the child. As Haldor Øvreeide and Reidun Hafstad point out, to develop, the child requires a hierarchical and asymmetrical distribution of responsibility between parents and child that is regulated to accommodate the child's needs and growing capacities. One implication of the child's dependence on adults is that it is virtually always the adults who define and articulate that the child has problems. The child, on the other hand, lives with the problem and expresses it from his or her own unique perspective, and, in many cases, the child's way of expressing the problem is seen by the adults as being the main problem.

In the therapeutic dialogue, it is essential to clarify both the difference in responsibility and the child's autonomy and capacities. It is in the field of tension between autonomy and independence that the child's development can unfold. For the child to develop through family therapy, the therapist, as a third party, should view his or her position as playing a limited and temporary role as a carer and, thus, becoming internalised as a new intrapsychic representation in the child. The therapist should promote a helpful dialogue between parents and child in order to help the parents understand and meet the child's needs in a responsible and developmentally supportive way (Figure 13). The experience of being seen and having his or needs

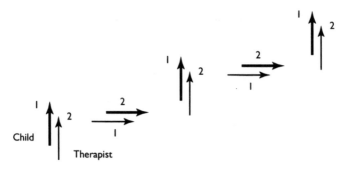

*Figure 13.* Following, leading, and adding in a developmental direction (source: Haldor Øvreeide's PowerPoint slides from the conference).

met will put the child in a position to express him/herself with greater clarity and confidence.

When adults show that they share the child's states, emotions, needs, and mental focus, the child responds. However, if the child fails to receive this form of synchronisation, his or development will be hampered. As Øvreeide points out, "sharing the mental state of the moment becomes the critical point in this kind of essential support . . . We become present in each other's states and needs. 'The other's' state becomes 'our own'" (Øvreeide, 2001, p. 25). By actively tuning in to the child, the adult becomes visible to the child. This lets the child become aware of both the adult's and his or her own states. An important aspect of the developmental process is to see oneself through someone else's eyes, which is what happens when the dialogic process opens up to allow mutually experienced present moments. The goal of the dialogue is to help the child achieve active mastery and the ability to look after his or her own and others' needs. The adult's recognition and guidance of the child in the attempts to master new areas of his or her zone of proximal development are a necessary condition for the child to develop social skills. For this to happen, there has to be a baseline level of appreciative intersubjective dialogic process between parents and child. Both children and adults are dependent on circular interactions of mutual appreciation in the healthy relationship, and it is central to the child's ability to realise his or her developmental potential.

Øvreeide (2001) points out that the therapeutic dialogue "has a dyadic process, but it virtually always also has triadic consequences" (p. 30). The therapist's task is to see and affirm the suffering the persons in the relationship are experiencing as well as their capacities and to make the individual's needs and competences visible to the significant others. The next step is for the therapist to notice, acknowledge, and, perhaps, challenge parental reactions to events and to support more adaptive ways of responding to the needs and states that are present in the child. The therapist's contributions to the dialogue should always contain elements of both affirmation and challenge in relation to the dependent person (the child) and the more responsible person (the parent).

Haldor Øvreeide summarises his treatment approach into five key factors that he believes the therapist should always keep in mind in interactions with children and parents.

1. The first factor is the child's *dependence*. The child expresses him/herself and matures in a continuous adaptation to someone who is bigger than the child.
2. The second factor is that *there are always inherent power issues*. The bigger person (the adult) is free to make choices and decisions, and it is, therefore, essential that his or her decisions match and accommodate the child's needs and stage of development. This power issue is important to keep in mind.
3. The third factor is *the co-operation process between the child and the parent or the therapist*. The child's ability to adapt and co-operate is a general and individual capacity that is present on all developmental stages and in all children.
4. The fourth factor is *meaning making*. As humans, we cannot interact with each other without perceiving the interaction as meaningful on some level. It is important to understand that meaning is created in the dyadic processes of relationships but is stored in the individual. Thus, the individual enters into the next situation with the stored meaning that is derived from the relationship.
5. Finally, the fifth key factor is that in interactions and relationships we are dyadic, but the dyadic communication always exists in a context of triadic and multiple relationships. We cannot communicate with another person without relating to the fact that there might be a third person who has a considerable interest in what is going on between the two persons in the dyad. This is an important reason for including the parents in the therapeutic process with children.

The developmentally supportive dialogue revolves around five key elements.

1. *Following*: the adult attunes with the child's physical and mental states—bodily, perceptually, emotionally, and cognitively.
2. *Relevance*: the adult stimulates curiosity by means of relevant information, emotional response, and structure.
3. *Agency space*: the adult provides time, physical and mental space, and recognition to accommodate and acknowledge the child's responses and build and support the child's self-organisation.
4. *Co-regulation*: the adult establishes rhythms and turn taking.
5. *Hierarchy*: the adult takes a lead position by embracing his or her overall responsibility and supportive intentions.

## Video clips from sessions presented
## at the conference by Haldor Øvreeide

### Therapy with Olaf

The mother that we see in this video brought Olaf in, and when I asked her if I could use this film in Copenhagen today, she said she would be very pleased if it might help others understand important things about children's development. The recordings were made two years ago, and today Olaf is living in a safe and well-supported relationship with his mother. But at this stage, some two years ago, this little family was in a crisis. The mother, whom I knew from before, had some traumatic childhood experiences, and she had been in therapy with me for some time. Now she was in a relationship with a man who was not Olaf's father, but she had cohabited with him for years, and Olaf sees him as his father. The stepfather had been using drugs for a while, and I think that for the last couple of years, the caring for Olaf had not been very good.

This culminated in an episode on Friday where the mother and stepfather got into a fight, the police had to come, and the ambulance had to come, and at this moment Olaf was taken into temporary foster care, so for two days now he has been staying with another family. But he comes in with his mother, together with some people from child protection, so that they could talk through what had happened on Friday. So that's the issue today, on Monday; they come here to talk through what happened on Friday. The mother is very tired at the moment; she has not slept, she says, for several days.

When Olaf came in, I said, "Welcome. You're coming here to talk with me and your mother, and we are going to talk here at the table while you are drawing."

*In the video, the mother looks at Haldor Øvreeide, while he sets up the video camera. At first, Olaf walks around, looking at things and taking in the room, as he has never been here before. This continues until Haldor Øvreeide says, "I need your help, Olaf, to set up the video."*

I include him in a project that might be of interest to him, and he's going to help me. So, in the lived moment, I try to be with the child and stay very close to his experience.

In the brief clip, we see how Haldor Øvreeide guides Olaf while also giving him time to calm down. Here, Haldor Øvreeide acted in the role of "caravan leader", clearly expressing a sense of calm and authority. He invited Olaf to engage in a co-operative and non-threatening activity instead of the small talk that is often used to kick off a session in therapy with adults. This behaviour supported Olaf's autonomic regulation, helped Olaf down-regulate his arousal level, and very quickly achieved the conditions for limbic affective attunement.

*In the video, Haldor Øvreeide shows Olaf what the video image looks like; Olaf checks it, and Haldor Øvreeide says, "Fine." "And then we will show me and you while I'm drawing," says Olaf. Haldor Øvreeide and Olaf sit down at the table. Olaf sits at the head of the table, while Haldor Øvreeide and the mother sit facing each other across the table. Olaf says, "But wait, wait, wait, we need a pencil." Haldor Øvreeide replies, "Yes, but I also wonder if you would like some apple juice or orange juice." Olaf replies, "I would like some apple juice. Can I go with you [to get it]?"*

> So, I give him structure, and within the structure I give him space to choose. And this is so amazing, when you provide a structure, and when you follow the lived moment of the child, the child very often falls into that structure and follows you. You have taken the lead, so here we see the principle of following, the principle of the hierarchy. So he follows. And the mother is sleeping while we are out [of the room].

Haldor Øvreeide supported the macro-regulation through micro-regulation and kindly offered Olaf some juice. Haldor Øvreeide always remained a small step ahead of Olaf with a clear idea of where he wanted to go. He supported his function as the person at the top of the power hierarchy, which made Olaf feel safe. Olaf accepted Haldor Øvreeide's superior position, and Haldor Øvreeide displayed caring and nurturing behaviour. He was letting Olaf know that "I am in control of what's happening; you can trust me, and I have good intentions for you."

*In the video, Haldor Øvreeide and Olaf have gone into the kitchen where they are helping each other find the bottle of apple juice. Olaf is not able to open the bottle, so Haldor Øvreeide says, "Your mother is strong." Initially, Olaf says, "No, she has just been in a fight." But then he changes his mind: "My mother can do it." Olaf and Haldor Øvreeide continue chatting about the project of getting the bottle open. Then they go into the therapy room, and*

*Olaf calls to his mother, who looks very tired. She seems depressed and passive and shows little reaction. Olaf says, "Mummy!" and tries to engage the mother, to lift her out of her non-responsive state. Haldor Øvreeide now says to the mother, "What have you told your boy today?"*

> Olaf and I were working together on finding the apple juice, but, as often as I can, I try to make this triangle, so that it's not only me and the child who co-operate. I try also to bring in the third party. So, here is a possibility to include the mother. Instead of me opening the bottle, Olaf now invites the mother in. So, moving along with the child with your body, the child will also experience the feeling of "Oh, I have a companion in my life." So you should signal this companionship.

> If I say, "What have you told Olaf," then I'm not giving them roles, but when I say, "What have you told your child, your boy, today?" I am giving the mother a role. In this situation, I am not sitting with Olaf and Hanna; I'm sitting with Olaf and his mother. Thus, I am using language to structure the relationship between the child and the carer.

*In the video, the mother says to Haldor Øvreeide, "I told him we were coming here to talk about what happened on Friday." Haldor Øvreeide says to Olaf, "I already know your mother from before," and Olaf says, "I would like to talk about it," and looks at his mother. Haldor Øvreeide says, "We can talk about whatever you like to talk about," and Olaf replies, "I want to talk about daddy." Olaf looks first at Haldor Øvreeide, then at his mother.*

> Why does he look at his mother? It's a question of power. We can see that he has something he wants to talk about, but he is unsure of the mother's response. We see two types of these glances in children. One type, which we are seeing here, expresses uncertainty, even anxiety: can I present myself, can I present my idea, or will it be rejected? It's a question of permission, and we can see that this has to do with the power part of the relationship. Then there is another glance, which is an intersubjective glance: are you experiencing what I am experiencing? We'll see if we can find some of those, too. But just at this moment, it's a question of permission or rejection.

*In the video, Olaf says, "You see, my mother doesn't want to live with my father any more." Haldor Øvreeide replies, "She does not want to live with him."*

> When the child says something, I repeat the expression, mirror it, so that the child can hear and register that I have taken it in. I want the

child to feel that I'm with him, and by repeating what the child is saying I am also helping the child to stay with his own initiative. The repetition supports his initiative. We see sometimes that clever parents are able to join in by naming what the child is expressing instead of asking additional questions. So, I register and help Olaf to stay with his initiatives.

In these repetitions, Haldor Øvreeide used marked mirroring, which let Olaf know, "I am feeling with you—I am able to follow you—I am interested in what you're thinking and feeling, and I have no problem containing what is happening." This function is important for achieving limbic attunement in a relationship with asymmetrical responsibility, which helps develop a space for Olaf to develop his mentalization capacity. As this is happening, Haldor Øvreeide also began to triangulate with the mother in order to facilitate her inclusion into the process.

*In the video, Haldor Øvreeide says, "You think that's OK that she doesn't . . ." and Olaf replies, "No." Haldor Øvreeide says, "So you want to live with him?" and Olaf says, "Yes, I want to . . ." Again, Olaf looks at his mother, a little uncertain. Haldor Øvreeide says, "You love your father." Now Olaf says, "Wait a moment." He gets up and goes over to check on the video camera, and the mother says, "No, stop!" Olaf says, "I just want to take a look," and the mother then says, "Come here." Haldor Øvreeide watches Olaf, follows him, and asks, "OK? Is it OK?" Olaf looks at Haldor Øvreeide, who smiles at him, and Olaf returns to the table.*

So Olaf breaks out, takes the initiative, and now we have a moment where we can analyse both the mother's and my own relationship with Olaf in this moment. The mother tries to stop Olaf, but, of course, he doesn't listen to her. And that's the problem; if there are more than ninety-five "stops", the child will ignore it. Then I try to help mother, "You're nervous," I say, and because I know her, that's OK. And then we just enjoy the moment for a while. But now we have introduced the questions.

*Haldor Øvreeide leaves the room to find some paper for drawing. He looks for a pencil and finds one. Then he says to Olaf, "If you turn your head" [Olaf turns his head as instructed] "you can see that are some pencils there, and you can take them."*

By describing the moment and describing his actions, I provide structure, and he carries out the action. But you can see how effective this is in helping him to concentrate on the moment. Because I describe the moment.

This is a boy who is very impulsive and active, and, by describing the moment, the lived moment, I help him to slow down and to get into his experiences, balancing his experience with his actions. I cannot stress enough how important this is, at least for me, when I want to help the child get into his own, to describe and share the lived moment. It is a very important way to help the child get into a structure or into a guiding process, so that we can get to the core of the therapy.

*In the video, Olaf begins to draw, occasionally looking up at his mother, who still appears very passive. Haldor Øvreeide says to Olaf, "So you don't think it's OK that your mother doesn't want to live with your father?" and Olaf replies, "No." The mother says that she has become afraid of the father, ". . . and it has been like that before." Haldor Øvreeide now tries to go into what happened in the incident on Friday and says to Olaf, "So on Friday . . . I think you had gone to bed?" Olaf looks away, then resumes eye contact with Haldor Øvreeide and says, "Yes." Haldor Øvreeide says, "On Friday night, you had gone to bed, and then you woke up because . . ." He stops and then continues, "And you woke up because of . . ." Olaf looks down at his drawing. He looks up, looks at Haldor Øvreeide, and then bursts out, "Don't you remember?!" as if he thinks that everybody must know what had happened. Haldor Øvreeide says, "No, I wasn't there." Olaf then says, "I dreamt yesterday. I dreamt a nightmare; I have nightmares, just like mummy has. She has some problems with . . ." Olaf looks at his mother. The mother responds with a little smile, and Haldor Øvreeide repeats Olaf's words. Olaf looks at Haldor Øvreeide, but then breaks off and does not want to talk about the nightmare any more. Instead, he says, "Can you help me draw a sunflower?" Haldor Øvreeide repeats, "A sunflower?" and Olaf says, "I want to show it to the camera." Again he looks at his mother, slightly nervous, as if he is saying, "Is this OK?" and Haldor Øvreeide replies warmly, "That's a good idea. We need green, and we need yellow . . ." Olaf gets out the paper and crayons, and Haldor Øvreeide suggests, "You can start with the yellow." He helps Olaf find the crayons, and Olaf draws. Then Haldor Øvreeide begins to talk, and Olaf interrupts: "Look at this!" as he shows off his drawing, then he says, "Five more minutes, OK?" Haldor Øvreeide nods, "OK."*

Haldor Øvreeide tried to guide the conversation with keywords to see if Olaf could be drawn into a dialogue about the traumatic incident while also allowing him to drift in and out of the topic. We saw how Haldor Øvreeide used marked mirroring and now added a narrative. At the same time, Olaf was focused on his mother, and Haldor Øvreeide was also aware of her role and presence. Olaf had associations to a sunflower that he remembered from home where he had lived with his mother and stepfather. Haldor Øvreeide supported this symbolisation and worked with the narrative in order to promote both Olaf's and his mother's mentalization.

> We have been in and a little out of the situation, and in a moment Olaf notices that his mother has received a text message on her phone. And then he has an idea.

> *In the video, Olaf says, "I want to call my daddy," and the mother says, "No, you can't, because the child protection service has said that you can't see your father for a long time. He has to stop taking drugs."*

> At this moment, the mother steps out of her role [as a mother] and says, "I'm a victim of circumstance, there's nothing I can do." Olaf goes into a state of despair. He can't stand the fact that he is not allowed to talk to his father. As you can see, I lean over towards the mother in a very intense way. I have a moral problem here, an ethical problem.

> *In the video, Haldor Øvreeide says, "Why can't he call his dad?! What kind of protection is that?!" Olaf gets up to check the camera. The mother buries her face in her hands. Olaf returns to the table and stands next to Haldor Øvreeide, who has pulled out a mobile phone. The mother says, "Sit down, Olaf, listen." Olaf stays with Haldor Øvreeide, who now takes charge and decides to call the stepfather from the therapy room. He gets the number from the mother, dials the number and says to Olaf, "And then you push this button." Olaf pushes the Call button, and thus, Olaf and Haldor Øvreeide work together to make the call.*

> Now we'll see what happens. Now the father might say, "Go to hell", we don't know, or maybe he won't pick up, but we are going into the world, trying to experience something about the situation together. We don't know what will happen.

*In the video, we hear the stepfather's voice in on the phone, and Haldor Øvreeide puts him on speaker. Olaf is intensely focused and asks, "Can I speak with him?" and Haldor Øvreeide says, "Yes. I'll just talk to him first." To the father, he says, "Good morning, it's the psychologist calling! I am talking to Olaf; it's good that you're awake. He wanted to hear your voice; he wanted to hear that you're OK." The stepfather asks, "Is it on loudspeaker?" and Haldor Øvreeide says, "Yes. Maybe you want to say something, Olaf?" Olaf is excited, he wipes his hands on his trousers, and says, "Hello, daddy!" and the stepfather replies, "Hi, my boy!" Olaf says, "Is my sunflower OK?" The stepfather hesitates . . . "The sunflower?" The mother smiles as she listens to this exchange. The stepfather now says, "Yes . . . I think so . . ." Haldor Øvreeide explains, "He is quite preoccupied with a sunflower. I understand that he has a sunflower. Are you at the house?" The stepfather says that he is, and Haldor Øvreeide asks him, "Could you just check on the sunflower?" The mother is smiling again. The stepfather goes outside to check on the sunflower and returns to say that it is fine, but it needs some water. After a few more exchanges, Olaf and his stepfather say goodbye and end the conversation.*

So, Olaf's idea about drawing a sunflower may have had a very important symbolic meaning to him: "It's my life, my old life, it's connected to the sunflower that I'm growing in my home." This is an experience I often have, that when you follow the unexpected initiatives of children when you are dealing with a troublesome area, very often these initiatives have some connection to the painful experience. Following the child's impulses will often lead you to the right or most precise moment.

Then I get a little moralistic; I say, "Things like that should not happen to a child," and both the mother and stepfather agree. So, sometimes, I step out of my role as a therapist. But parents very often second that, of course, both because morals are like that, and also, if we had the time, you could see that these were, in fact, deep-felt responsibilities for both the mother and the stepfather.

*In the video, Haldor Øvreeide and the mother now talk about the stepfather and the family history. Meanwhile, Olaf has drawn a red heart that he wants to send to his stepfather to tell him, "I still love you." Haldor Øvreeide asks the mother if she wants to draw something too, and she draws a broken heart.*

We are building a narrative that takes in his experience and his feelings for his father and mother at this moment, but also a more realistic part of the story, of the conditions that they live under, that the stepfather has to stop using drugs before he can enter into a relationship with Olaf.

This sequence continued to explore symbolisation and reality testing, as Olaf's feelings of love were given space and recognition alongside both the stepfather's drug addiction and the mother's pain. This work supported an ongoing processing of the situation and a higher level of mentalization, which are functions related to the maturation of prefrontal processes.

*In the video, Olaf now brings in an envelope and a stamp. The mother says, "Oh, you have an envelope." Olaf hands it to her, and she says, "Yes, we can do that." Together, they open the envelope, put in the letter with Olaf's drawings, pull off the strip and seal the envelope. Haldor Øvreeide says to Olaf, "Mummy will show you how. Mummy will write the name and address." Olaf looks very pleased. He is now sitting on the mother's side of the table; they are co-operating and engaging in joint attention.*

The process between Olaf and his mother is now much more supportive. They are co-operating, they have a product now.

*In the video, Olaf asks his mother to write, "From Olaf to daddy", and Haldor Øvreeide says, "Yes, that's right, and inside it says that you love him." Olaf replies, "And my heart is there." Haldor says, "And you have a heart that is not broken." Olaf says, "I don't have a heart that is broken, like mummy's. Like this." Olaf holds up his mother's drawing. Haldor says, "Yes, mummy's heart is broken a little." Olaf then gets up, stands next to his mother, bends over and listens to her heart. "I want to listen."*

Olaf is not quite certain that his mother's heart is broken. I would like to reflect a little on this moment, because for me, this is a now moment with the mother. We can see that the mother has a positive look on her face; she is looking at me, and we are sharing our joy over Olaf. In this moment, we can be certain that the mother has taken her child in, and that her feelings for him are what a mother's feelings should be. I think that this moment was very important for the mother, when they made this distinction between the mother's feelings for the father and the child's feelings, and she accepted Olaf as a self-experiencing subject in the situation.

From this moment, for the next two years, she has been doing very well with Olaf, taking much more initiative to protect him, and she also wanted to work with Reidun. She knew that we work with Marte Meo, and Reidun did a couple of sessions with Marte Meo, helping the mother to lead and structure the daily processes with Olaf.

## Summary

This chapter describes a therapy process that linked the limbic and the prefrontal compass. Olaf had undergone a traumatic experience, and his mother also appeared traumatised, unable to provide relevant protection and meet him in his longing for the stepfather, whom he was not allowed to see. The therapy process was characterised by a triadic approach to Olaf's attachment process with the mother and support for mentalizing narratives and reality-testing. Haldor Øvreeide used his therapeutic position to provide structure in a developmentally supportive way. He offered a structured path for Olaf with proposals that the boy was able to follow, but the structure also clearly gave Olaf influence and acknowledged his suggestions. In doing this, Haldor Øvreeide served as a role model for the mother, modelling ways for an adult to support a child and act as the child's advocate. Haldor Øvreeide used the symbolism of the heart to define a distinction between Olaf and his mother and an acceptance of their separate positions in relation to Olaf's stepfather. Olaf's development of prefrontal capacities remains fragile. This is evident both in his lack of understanding that Haldor Øvreeide had not been present during the violent episode, corresponding to difficulties on the axis of ego-altercentric participation in the limbic compass, and in his inadequate sense of object permanence (for example, when he failed to understand that the stepfather could not see the drawing of a sunflower that he had just made). Haldor Øvreeide supports the mentalizing process by leading, following, and contributing, both in action sequences and by means of narratives with symbolic content.

# CHAPTER SIX

# The second growth spurt and multi-family mentalization-based therapy

"The first step in the treatment process is to make the problem concrete and present in the actual context. This contextual approach means that if people have an eating problem, we want to see how they eat; if people have a sleeping problem, we go to their house at bedtime; and if the child has problems in school, we come to the school, etc. This means that the work of the clinic not only takes place at the clinic but also in the context where the problem unfolds"

(Asen)

In this chapter, we address the second growth spurt, looking at the more sophisticated forms of mentalization, which mature gradually from around two years after birth until after adolescence, and the neural structures that we consider essential during this growth spurt. Next, we discuss multi-family mentalization-based therapy, an approach developed by the German child psychiatrist, Eia Asen, and his colleagues at the Marlborough Family Service in London.

*Second growth spurt and the maturation of the prefrontal level*

As we saw in the previous chapter, the first growth spurt involves the brain's basic activation on all levels and, thus, also the development of the child's basic being in the body, in the world, and in a safe and caring dyadic relationship. The second growth spurt is about linking language to one's self-sense and to the outside world, developing biographical narratives, and increasing degrees of autonomy in relation to one's family, the maturation of the mentalization capacity, forming equal relationships, and the ability to enter flexibly into a wide variety of groups of varying size and complexity.

This long phase lasts from the age of two years until the early twenties and includes the main development of the reflective mentalization capacity. The simple, or primitive, mentalization capacity is formed by the interlinking of important internal representations through the development of neural networks, forming more coherent and complex mental images in connection with the limbic structures. During the first period of the second growth spurt, the limbic areas develop or reorganise; this means that the formation of representations is mediated primarily by the brain's emotional association areas. This process gradually results in the formation of coherent representations of self, significant others, and the world at large. Later in this phase, as our sense of time, logical and causal thinking, and our capacity for empathy develop, the formation of representations is tied more closely to neural structures in the neocortex. The myelinisation of more highly developed brain regions leads to a replacement of primitive behaviour by volitional acts. This is a gradual process, as the areas that co-ordinate behaviour and attention are not fully myelinated until after puberty. In the next section, we offer an overview of the development of the brain during the second growth spurt before moving on to a discussion of maturation-specific themes during this period.

*Brain maturation during the second growth spurt*

Both the first and the second growth spurt are completed with a process of pruning and parcellation. Thus, there are some similarities in the final stages of the two growth spurts, at the age of two years and the end of adolescence, respectively, and both periods play a formative role in our personality development. In the course of childhood and youth, the surface of the cortex becomes increasingly folded up to make room for the twenty billion neurons in the adult brain (Gjærum & Ellertsen, 2002; Trevarthen, 1990). The second growth spurt marks a period of unparalleled selection and sophistication in the neocortical connections that form the basis of conscious processes in the prefrontal system. From the age of two years until adolescence, it is especially the shorter neural connections that mature; this increases the degree of nuance and functional capacity in the individual areas and in the connections with adjacent areas (Fair, Cohen, Power, et al., 2009; Supekar, Musen, & Menon, 2009). From the age of seven years until adulthood, the brain's neural networks go from mainly being organised in small circuits involving adjacent areas to being organised in systems that co-ordinate far-flung areas into functional circuits, which is believed to improve precision and regulation in the brain's higher functions (Fair, Cohen, Power, et al., 2009). As in the first major growth spurt, the change processes during the second growth spurt occur mainly in specific parts of the brain during specific periods, and neurophysiologists associate these growth periods with important phases of cognitive development (Chamley, Carson, & Randall, 2005).

## The dorsolateral prefrontal cortex

The most important development during this phase is the maturation of the dorsolateral prefrontal cortex, which is situated in the exterior side of the back of the prefrontal cortex. The dorsolateral prefrontal cortex is the most important structure for co-ordinating external information and internal reactions as well as for co-ordinating and focusing emotional and cognitive impressions and planning actions. It is this area that enables us to hold and manipulate mental images, and this is where plans and ideas take shape. It enables us to choose one strategy over another and arrive at carefully considered emotional responses. Among other functions, it serves to suppress or control emotions to enable us to respond more effectively to a given situation or initiate a new response if a re-assessment indicates that one is needed. The dorsolateral prefrontal cortex is a key structure in our working memory and enables us to hold a piece of information long enough to manipulate it mentally. This area enables us to organise and reorganise; it is the seat of our ability to resist distractions and urges to respond prematurely. This is the area that inhibits impulses or behaviours that are deemed inappropriate.

Although the dorsolateral prefrontal cortex and the orbitofrontal cortex are situated side by side, their neural circuits, biochemistry, and functions are very different. Both the dorsolateral prefrontal cortex and the orbitofrontal cortex are important for inhibition and control, but while the dorsolateral areas are more involved in conscious decision-making processes, the decision-making processes in the orbitofrontal cortex rely more on affective information. While the orbitofrontal cortex plays an important role in implicit behaviour regulation, the dorsolateral prefrontal cortex is essential for explicit behaviour regulation. For example, explicit behaviour regulation lets us correct our behaviour, to some extent, when we become aware that we have acted inappropriately, while implicit behaviour regulation occurs on a preconscious level. The dorsolateral prefrontal cortex allows us to be mentally present both in the here and now and, simultaneously, somewhere else. Our attention goes wherever our thoughts go. When experiences are put into a context of time and place, the dorsolateral prefrontal cortex is activated. The dorsolateral prefrontal cortex plays an important role in our ability to recall sequential memories. The area has to be capable of multi-tasking and of switching rapidly among cognitive tasks. Information has to be brought into focus as needed, and we need to be able to switch rapidly between fields of relevant information (Goldberg, 2001).

## The maturation of the higher levels of mentalization

Many of the developmental skills that we need to acquire between the age of two years and adulthood are unique to humans. During this long developmental phase, the emotional learning capacities that have developed on the basis of the autonomic and the limbic system need to be tied more closely into the prefrontal system and sophisticated cognitive processes. This includes the ongoing development of object constancy, the capacity for attention control and reality testing, role-playing and symbolic play, the development of narratives, symbolisation, and the reflective function (mentalization capacity), the capacity for perspective-taking and the development of feelings of shame, conscience, and morality.

While social learning during the first growth spurt relied mainly on the infant's interactions with carers and other family members, during the second growth spurt, from the age of two years into the mid-twenties, the child and, later, the teenager relates both to the parents and to other adult authority figures, such as teachers and leaders of after-school activities, who serve as role models. Increasingly, the child also takes part in shaping subcultures and ways of being with peers. During childhood and youth, the child develops close relations and friendships with peers in both dyadic contacts and groups. Within the framework of these relations, the child builds on and develops the contact skills, attachment forms, and behavioural and interaction norms he or she acquired in the family context. In the following, we look at the specific competences that develop during the second growth spurt.

## The development of object constancy

Internal representations are shaped by the child's history, and, as the brain matures and object constancy develops, the child becomes able to maintain internal representations outside the original situation. Internal representations are a form of internalisation process, where intersubjective relations become intrasubjective. One example might be the internalisation of the emotional experience of being praised or humiliated by one's father or mother. The child forms internal representations from within and contributes his or her own interpretation and subjective experience of the interaction, and this can be addressed and processed in psychotherapy. For example, the child might have a stern internal representation that has become internalised through representations of relationships with the child as an active participant. Our internal representations contribute to our understanding of the world, make our world more predictable, and are crucial in all our future relationships, but they can be influenced and reshaped in subsequent relationships.

During the first seven to nine months after birth, the child depends on the carer's presence for self-regulation. It is only as the maturation of the orbitofrontal cortex produces object constancy that the child begins to be able to maintain internal representations of the interaction with the carer, even when she is not present. Object constancy is initiated around the age of seven months, but is not fully developed until the age of three years. As the child's emergent object constancy develops, the child enjoys playing with the permanence of things, for example, in the game of "peekaboo". At the age of seven to nine months, the child begins to be able to move around independently, and, thanks to object constancy, objects are no longer "out of sight, out of mind" (Emde, 1989; Sroufe, 1989; Stern, 1977, 1985).

With the development of the orbitofrontal area, the child begins to experience continuity of past, present, and future. The child is able to sustain interactions over time, which means engaging in relationships, and, at this time, a disturbance in the contact between the child and the carer will begin to be evident as a relational disorder, which the child also brings into other relationships. The internal representation that replaces the carer when she is not present helps the child achieve impulse inhibition and self-soothing. However, it may also act as an internalised phenomenon that inhibits the child's activities and expression, which might need to be addressed and processed in psychotherapy. The child begins to be able to establish transitional objects to aid self-regulation and provide emotional soothing by mimicking the interaction with the carer. By establishing internal representations of the carer, the child is able to maintain a mental image of her that helps guide the child's behaviour (Bråten, 1993). Once this capacity has been established, a psychotherapist may also represent an important transitional object for the child until a caring and nurturing other is internalised.

While the ability to sustain mental images is established around the age of twelve months, the capacity for building mental representations of others' mental representations does not emerge until the age of eighteen months. This marks yet one more step on the path to developing the type of object constancy that will not be in place until much later, which involves perceiving oneself and others as constant entities, regardless of one's own or the other's present mood or feeling. The capacity for building mental representations of others' mental representations further develops the child's self-boundaries, as the child is now able to distinguish between his or her own and others' experiences and internal representations. The child begins to develop a sense of how he or she is perceived by others and to be able to understand things from another's perspective; both of these abilities are key components of the mentalization capacity.

## Role-playing and symbolic play

At the age of two years, the child begins to interact more with peers, and by the time he or she reaches four years of age, the child has begun to establish friendship relations through mutual role-playing and to prefer certain children over others. The child's capacity for play develops and, from parallel play, the child now begins to engage in shared play, which unfolds in a reciprocal process. There is evidence to suggest a link between the child's ability to assess and understand others' thoughts and the child's experiences with shared pretend play. Children's social understanding develops as a result of conflict resolution situations, where they have to include others' points of view in negotiations, and as a result of recurring experiences with sharing, arguing, and negotiating with others in a pretend world where they are confronted with other children's varying perspectives and points of view. In addition to turn-taking, these skills also include things like being able to share toys and other assets, engaging in joint attention in play, incorporating others' ideas in play, agreeing on ground rules, resolving conflicts, and making up after fights. All these skills are trained in the asymmetrical relations with carers and other adults, and they are stabilised through peer experiences with other children in symmetrical interactions.

## The development of the reflective function

From around the age of three to four years, children begin to be able to reflect on other people's mental states. This expanded mentalization capacity makes it possible to assess one's own and others' mental models, to plan activities and to assess, re-assess, and predict events. The child's social understanding also develops through conversations about emotions and mental states, especially with the child's carers (Dunn, 1996). This forms an early foundation for the shift from a self-centred reality to a perception of the self as embedded in a larger whole that the individual co-creates, which one both nourishes and is nourished by.

Around the age of 4–5 years, the child develops the ability to draw causal conclusions and to connect related representations over time. The integration of the parietal areas and the limbic system with the orbitofrontal and dorsolateral prefrontal cortex combines our emotional and our cognitive intelligence, which forms the basis for reflective mentalization. Here, the cognitive integration and the emergence of a mentalization capacity are crucial elements. Thanks to the child's mentalization capacity, other people's actions become meaningful and predictable, which, in turn, reduces the child's dependence on others. The dorsolateral prefrontal cortex continues to develop, and the capacity for attention control that this area enables lets the child focus his or her attention as needed and master adaptive behaviour inhibition. The capacity for directed control also enables the child to engage in psychological intimacy, which involves the ability to sense another person's feelings and thoughts without being overwhelmed by the other's suffering or discomfort. If this capacity is inadequate, the child is either overwhelmed or feels compelled to distance him/herself from the other's pain. This is an important step in the child's individuation process.

The mentalization capacity enables the child not only to react to another person's behaviour, but also to act on his or her concepts of others' assumptions, emotions, attitudes, wishes, hope, knowledge, and imagination. It enables the child to "read" other people mentally. The child's previous experiences with others make it possible to establish and structure multiple sets of self- and other-representations (Fonagy et al., 2007).

Mentalization is predominantly an implicit (unconscious) function, like riding a bicycle. However, only when the capacity is fully developed does mentalization become an ongoing process, as the child seeks constantly to understand and respond to other people's wishes, expectations, and feelings, both in order to influence their behaviour and in order to attune with them. This expanded mentalization makes it possible to understand and predict other people's behaviour, and the self-reflecting function makes the child's behaviour more intelligent. The child's ability to influence his or her own actions rely on the child's ability to process and reflect on his or her own and other's feelings, actions, wishes, etc. (Fonagy et al., 2000), which requires mature prefrontal symbolising and verbal competences. If feelings remain unsymbolised, for example if the child is unable to recognise and express feelings of anger or fear by talking about them or perhaps drawing an angry or frightened face, the child will not be able to process the feelings explicitly (consciously). In that case, the feelings are either acted out, for example, through aggressive behaviour or self-harming behaviour, or expressed in psychosomatic symptoms, as the child lacks the ability to process his or her emotions on a mental, reflective level (Gerhardt, 2004).

The development of the ability to relate with empathy both to oneself and to others, the ability to see oneself and others in a greater interpersonal perspective, and the ability to make realistic plans refine and promote the development of the prefrontal cortex and its regulation of limbic and autonomic affective processes. Reality testing and support for accepting and assimilating both pleasant and unpleasant feelings are essential aspects of therapy at this level. Other well-known themes in the therapeutic exchange are the difficulty in understanding the other's perspective and in understanding that not all wishes, whether one's own or others', can be fulfilled. Being able to reflect on an incident or one's own personality is no good if it does not lead to modifications of the feelings and narratives associated with these incidents or qualities. That sort of "unconnected" reflection capacity may be described as pseudo-mentalization, as the child might appear to engage in reflective processing but is, in fact, merely expressing a new, unreflected narrative.

### Coherent memories and perspective taking

Around the age of three to four years, the child begins to be able to tie memories into a coherent structure of time and shape narratives around them, which leads to the establishment of an autobiographical self. Fonagy and colleagues (2007) point out that the ability to link multiple related representations over time creates the basis for establishing an abstract historical self-concept that integrates memories of different self-states that can be articulated verbally. From the age of six to seven years, symbols become more important and useful in the intuitive sharing of information around an interpreted reality. This is the stage when the child begins to be able to relate to him/herself on a mental level. Both as children and as adults, we rely on our capacity for empathy to reflect on ourselves. It is only by seeing ourselves through someone else's eyes that we can become aware, on a higher mental level, that we have a self that is separate from another's self. This ability to see ourselves from the other's point of view is also at the heart of our ability to form stable friendships and romantic relationships, which is a recurring theme in psychotherapy. In order to understand why our relationships are the way they are, we need to be able to see ourselves from the other's perspective.

## The development of narratives and the capacity for abstraction and symbolising

When the child develops language, that facility may replace physical acts, just as we can also use language to exchange ideas and plans and to move or thrill each other (Rizzolatti & Arbib, 1998). The language that we use for mentalization and self-reflection reflects a level of integration where sensations and affects are integrated, making it possible for us to have thoughts about emotions. In healthy self-reflection, emotions are associated with an explicit understanding that is capable of editing our narratives about who we are and of building mentalized interpersonal connections. When the child's autonomic and limbic areas have matured, the child will use narrative processes to make sense of the world and co-ordinate his or her own internal states. Sometimes, the child will also use narratives as a means of cognitive self-reflection.

Narrative processes and therapy forms based on narratives are a real option only with adults, whose arousal and affect regulation competences have matured to a level where verbal statements can be used to modify the person's internal environment. If these therapeutic approaches are used with children whose basic personality competences have not yet matured, the child will simply revert to previous emotional, cognitive, and action patterns after the completion of the therapeutic process.

From the age of seven years, the child is able to form higher cognitive abstractions and symbols. At the age of 7–13 years, the child begins to develop a real capacity for hypothesising, understanding probabilities, forming ideals, and testing possibilities. Towards the end of this age span, the more mature forms of identity formation begin to emerge in the form of a capacity for self-reflection, self-objectification, interpreting social contexts, and choosing strategies and social roles. The child's thinking becomes more logical, and the child is able to enter into varying roles, drawing on countless simultaneous perspectives. The development of the child's self-image at this age level requires the understanding that we are involved in both constructing and interpreting our own history (Fonagy et al., 2007; Frønes, 1994; Hobson, 1993; Neisser, 1993; van der Kolk, 1987). Identity formation at this stage relies on the capacity for reflective mentalization, and, generally, the child's own identity is taking clearer shape at this time.

At the age of twelve years, the child obtains much greater insight into his or her own emotions, and cognitive reflection enables the child to develop internal representations, which may be mutually contradictory and ambivalent. The child is no longer limited to addressing a single aspect of a problem and is able to draw on countless simultaneous perspectives, also in his or her relations with others. At this age level, the child is able to distinguish clearly between perceived reality and fantastical (or deceptive) narratives that are governed by wishful thinking and a search for social affirmation from oneself and others and to relate to different aspects of his or her own personality. The child becomes increasingly able to consider the intention behind actions and to relate to conflicted emotions towards others (Øvreeide, 2002; Tetzchner, 2002).

## The development of guilt, conscience, and morality

As described in the previous chapter, shame pertains to the child's being and is a condition for the later development of guilt. Guilt does not develop until after the child has acquired language. The two-to-four-year-old child is still self-centred and experiences the world as revolving around him or her, but this means not only that the child is the world champion, it also means that the child is to blame when something goes wrong. During the second year of life, the child begins to be able to distinguish between right and wrong (Bruner, 1990). As early as at the age of two and a half years, the child might begin to deny having done something wrong, even when the child is obviously culpable. The child also begins to be able to adapt his or her behaviour:

for example, by concealing emotions that he or she has learnt are un-acceptable in order to avoid criticism and insensitive reactions from others. As the child's mental and cognitive capacities develop, the child is better able to present cogent arguments, even when he or she is angry or sad, and the child strives for self-understanding and for solving problems that arise in a social context. The child finds ways to co-operate with others and gain their approval, which enhances the child's self-esteem. At an early stage, the child is also focused on comparing his or her own capabilities and achievements to those of others and is actively engaged in constructing rules and morals. Guilt requires awareness of the concept of norms and an understanding that others demand compliance with these norms. This understanding later forms part of the basis for the development of morality. Similarly, a sense of embarrassment requires a sense of how other people might judge one's behaviour, which, in turn, requires imagination (Øvreeide, 2002; Rutter & Rutter, 1997; Sroufe, 1979; van der Kolk, 1987).

The ability to see oneself through the eyes of others may activate the sense of shame, which is status-related, as the child becomes pre-occupied with the way in which others perceive the child and his or her family. The shame associated with looking bad is an important issue for many people, children as well as adults, and often forms the core of narratives from children and adults.

Around the age of nine to ten years, the child becomes increasingly aware that other people's feelings are not only affected by the conse-quences of the child's actions, but also by the feelings and non-verbal reactions that the actions trigger in others. Pride and guilt become key phenomena, not only as a result of other people's judgement, but also as a result of the child's own internal sense of responsibility. At the age of eight to ten years, the child begins to develop a conscience, which means that the child begins to be able to attribute a negative emotion to his or her own actions and to assess his or her own intentionality: for example, when the child feels guilty about his or her thoughts about others.

## The second growth spurt and child psychotherapy

In many cases, it is an inadequate capacity for mental images and mentalization that forms the underlying issue when parents are locked into a conflict with their child, have negative expectations of the child and their surroundings, are unable to take the child's perspective, view the child as the source of the problem, or attribute a conflict to an inherent flaw in the child without being able to relate to themselves, and the child is locked into maladaptive reactions. Reality testing and support with accepting and assimilating both pleasant and unpleasant emotions are key aspects of therapy, especially in relation to the parents, but also in relation to the slightly older child.

Effective mentalization depends on the connection with the previously matured deeper layers of the personality. One cannot truly reflect on an incident or on one's own personality unless the reflection changes one's feelings or narratives. As described above, such an "unconnected" reflection capacity would constitute pseudo-mentalization, as the person appears to engage in reflective processing, while, in fact, merely relating a more rational-sounding, unreflected narrative. When the parents or the slightly older child are unable to apply their prefrontal, causal thinking and find that the unpleasant experiences keep repeating themselves, they are missing out on the opportunity to achieve a different outcome and of examining the impact of other possible courses of action.

When the child acquires language, narratives take on a structuring function for one's self-concept. The integration of the non-verbal and the verbal level is important for developing a sense of self, a self-organising capacity, and, thus, psychological resilience. However, the danger of a verbal narrative is that what is captured in words will always differ from the original non-verbal experience, and that the verbal representation of the self, which is primarily situated in the left brain hemisphere, may therefore be separate and detached from the bodily and emotional representation, which is situated mainly in the right brain hemisphere. This is a distinction that is rarely drawn in psychotherapy.

The internalisation of norms and requirements that activate the sense of guilt is related to the psychological component that we called the "archaic superego" in the discussion of the prefrontal compass model in the previous chapter. Much psychotherapeutic work is focused on how the archaic superego became an integrated part of the parents' or the child's self-concept, and how the psychotherapy process can enable the person to identify and break off from the undigested superego introjects that create a conflict with the being in various emotional categories that develop the limbic structures, which, in turn, are a source of confidence and inner calm. In many cases, the introjected superego is perceived as a deprecating, scolding, brutal judge. Like shame, guilt is a severe affective dysregulation that has become an intrapsychological structure, and, in the effort to create reflective levels of mentalizations, the child or the parents need help from an authority figure to regulate out of the unpleasant feeling and, next, to establish a regulatory internal authority that is capable of containing the archaic superego. The more nuanced understanding depends on the capacity to contain and regulate, and the parents or the child first need help to establish an internal perspective that contains both the internal authority figure that assigns the guilt and the person who feels driven by this feeling of guilt.

Now, we look at a therapeutic method, multi-family mentalization-based therapy, which was developed by Eia Asen and others at the Marlborough Family Service in London.

## Multi-family mentalization-based therapy by Eia Asen

At the time of the conference, Eia Asen worked both at the Marlborough Family Service and at the Anna Freud Centre, both of which were located in central London. (As we mentioned earlier in the book, he now works only at the Anna Freud Centre, but we will let his words stand in the present tense in the following, in order to be representative of when they were spoken.) Asen explains that the Marlborough Family Service is a very busy place that works with families from all over the world, who often present multiple problems at once. With a therapeutic staff of forty-five, many of them part-time, the clinic takes in about 1,000 new cases a year. This caseload makes it necessary to come up with creative methods to be able to keep up with demand, and it was through the close co-operation with the Anna Freud Centre that the staff at the Marlborough Family Service became interested in working with a mentalization-based approach.

Eia Asen explains that since the place is called "Marlborough" he will stick to the letter M to describe the multi-family mentalization-based method. He then goes on to describe the Marlborough model as a multi-contextual, multi-systems, multi-cultural, multi-modal, multi-mentalizing, and multi-family approach! Multi-contextual means that they look at the child or the person in a given context: in the family context, in the friendship context, in the school context, if it is a child, in the larger neighbourhood and cultural context (Figure 14). This also includes the larger context of the helping system, because many of the families the centre works with have multiple helpers. Asen mentions that the record so far is fifty-six helpers for one family—social workers, support persons, etc.

Work at the Marlborough Family Service is primarily family-systemic and multi-family based; in addition, they also do a fair amount of social networking. In their work, the therapists usually rely on parallel interventions at many different levels. They work not only with the child, but often also include the parents and the rest of the family as well as networks of friends. As many of the families they work with have close ties to their religious community, for example, the mosque, the temple, the synagogue, or the church, they often

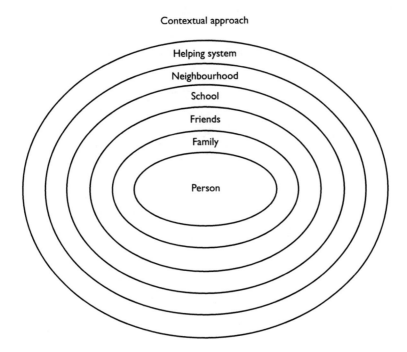

Contextual approach

Helping system
Neighbourhood
School
Friends
Family

Person

*Figure 14.*   Contextual approach
(source: Eia Asen's PowerPoint slides from the conference).

include community leaders (Figure 15). The religious leaders are important helpers in the systemic work. The centre employs Islamic counsellors in an effort to make the work acceptable to all cultures.

The Marlborough Family Service does not have a marketed, protected, specific brand of therapy—as Eia Asen says, tongue-in-cheek, "We steal from everybody. We also invent some ideas. So, for different people, we do different things." Often, the therapists will place a family in a group with other families, so that six to ten families are together for hours or days at a time, often over a period of several weeks or months. They use this approach for a number of reasons: one is that it might be easier for the family members to observe issues with attachment, relationships, connections, projections, etc., in other families than in their own. It also lets the families support and engage each other and share their difficulties. They can offer each other hope and encourage change, they can observe and challenge each other's family patterns, and they can share strategies and explore behavioural changes. The multi-family group approach is very helpful when the families take part in an open or running group where they can meet

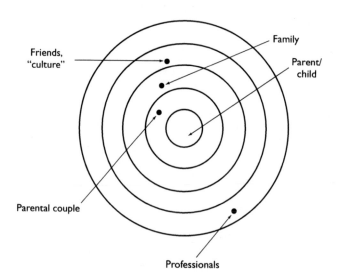

Figure 15.    Levels and contexts for the intervention
(source: Eia Asen's PowerPoint slides from the conference).

other families with similar issues to their own. For example, the Marlborough Family Service has multi-family groups for children with ADHD, Asperger's syndrome, etc. Often, the multi-family approach helps the parents to see themselves in a new light. It helps the families to see that they are not the only ones who have a given problem, but that other families are facing similar challenges. The multi-family approach helps the families escape isolation and stigmatisation, compare experiences, and see themselves mirrored in others. This lets them move from helplessness to helpfulness and establish social connections with each other.

The first step in the treatment process is to make the problem concrete and present in the actual context. This contextual approach means that if people have an eating problem, the therapists want to see how they eat; if people have a sleeping problem, therapists go to their house around bedtime; if the child has problems in school, they go to the school, etc. Thus, the work not only takes place at the clinic, but also in the context where the problem unfolds.

As there is limited time available for each family, the therapist usually sees four or five families at the same time. For example, one therapy room might have a family where a child has an eating problem, and the therapist will ask the family to start their meal and then return later to see how they are getting on. In another room, there might be a mother who has a child who has problems getting his homework done, and they are asked to begin doing homework. And so forth. All the rooms have one-way mirrors, and the therapist moves between the rooms, observes through the mirror to develop a sense of what is going on, and then enters the room to introduce a brief intervention. The family therapist may deliberately choose to create a crisis as part of the intervention: for example, by making unexpected demands. Stress patterns show up very clearly in crisis situations, and it is by addressing these patterns that people can discover new possible ways of acting. The therapy team works within a mentalization-based framework and records therapy situations on video, as video recordings are very useful in helping people reflect on their own and others' reactions and intentions. The recordings of the deliberately introduced crisis situations are later used to reflect, with the family, after they have calmed down and have some distance to the incident—a week, a year, or half an hour later. In this reflection process, the family therapist goes from being a directive therapist who presents a range of tasks and makes demands to being a mentalizing therapist, who, instead, says things such as, "Why do you think your father does that?" The key to mentalizing interventions is to preserve one's own curiosity and to invite the family members to join the therapist in wondering and looking for explanations.

### Video clips from multi-family mentalization-based therapy sessions presented at the conference by Eia Asen

#### Therapy with Akil

I'll introduce you to this boy. He's called Akil, and we're going to follow him and his family to look at specific and, above all, non-specific factors that one can use, perhaps, across all the modalities of work in psychotherapy. So, this is a boy, a typical boy. In England, people are not as mad on diagnoses as they are in Sweden, and not quite as bad as in Denmark, but still, most of our children have a lot of diagnoses. Usually two, three, or four. It's usually ADHD or autistic spectrum disorder or, if the child swears and says "shit" and other, worse words, they get the label Tourette's on top of that. And if their emotions go up and down, they're called bipolar disorder of childhood, or even infancy. Akil only has two diagnoses—I thought I'd pick an easy case ... But in school he's very cut off, he has no friends, he's distracted, and he's very irritable, he can never focus on anything; he's disruptive and under-functioning academically. At home, he's a huge problem. He's an only child, and he doesn't eat. If he does eat something, it takes him three or four or five hours. He's a very anxious child; he has to sleep in the mother's bed, he cannot be alone in the room by himself, he's very demanding, very babyish—these are the words of the parents.

The parents run a restaurant, and the father works most of the time, also nights. Akil had a very difficult birth; he was premature and was in an incubator for ten weeks. He nearly died. The mother had huge health problems as well, so for the first year of his life he had a pretty rough time. The parents are Turkish and Iraqi, they've been in England for five years, for political reasons.

Our sessions are usually between ten minutes and half an hour, and the parents and the boy decide that the first issue they're going to tackle is the eating, because the parents have said the eating is the biggest problem. After the initial telephone conversation the parents have decided that all three of them will come in for the first session. So, they come in with a huge, problem-saturated narrative: ". . . and he does that, and he does that . . ." Akil just sat there, and he was distracted, he was all over the place. Just listened to it. So I will show you the second session now, where it's only the mother together with Akil.

*In the video, we see Akil seated at a table with an array of little bowls of food. He is picking at the food with his fork, dropping some of it and coughing when he puts a tiny bite in his mouth; meanwhile his mother watches with a look of grave concern.*

And his mother is a wonderful mother, she cooks food, beautiful food, and she's brought three courses, and all the three courses are already out there, and he's hardly eaten any of it. So here's some soup, which the mother had cooked. Six hours she cooked that incredibly nourishing soup! And he just picks at it. Can you imagine what goes through this poor mother's mind—and this in public!

Through the one-way screen, I see this happening: I see how he messes around and talks to his mother. He's meant to be eating, but she talks to him, and he responds, and he eats a little bit or nothing. He usually takes the food out of his mouth, then puts it back. I'm behind the one-way screen; I'm much less patient than the mother. You'll see it in a minute. By the way, I have to warn you, the intervention you're about to see here is shocking. Prepare yourselves! It's not made for the Danish context. There's no candles, there's nothing *hyggelig* [nice and cosy] about it! He talks some garbage, and the mother talks to him, and then I come into the room.

*In the video, Eia Asen enters the room and says to Akil, "What are you doing?" Akil replies, "Eating." Eia Asen: "Eating? Could have fooled me! How is it going? Is it going well?" The mother answers, "Yes, we are doing well." Eia Asen leaves the room after indicating that he is going to watch through the one-way mirror. Akil puts a little bit of food in his mouth but then waves his mother over. The mother says, "No, you can eat by yourself," and Akil replies, "No, I can't." The mother asks, "Are you a baby?" and Akil replies, "Yes!!" The mother says, "Oh, do you want mummy to feed you now?" Akil pushes the food away, and the mother says, "Oh, because mummy's not feeding you?! But you're a big boy now!" and Akil says, "I don't want food." The mother says, in mock anger, "But you said you were hungry. You're lying to me now!!" Eia Asen enters the room again.*

That's enough for me! A very specific intervention is required!

*In the video, Eia Asen says to the mother, "Why don't you go out now, mummy, and you come back when he's finished." Eia Asen then turns to Akil: "Mummy will come back when you've finished." Akil: "What!" "She will come back when you've finished. If you don't finish, she won't come back."*

Wow! I wouldn't like to say it again like that, but I'm showing you all my tapes, as we say in England, 'warts and all', all the crap as well, which you can comment on; my non-specific crap.

*In the video, Eia Asen and the mother leave the room, closing the door behind them. Akil throws himself off the chair, screaming loudly, and runs wailing to the door, banging on it. "I'm dying!!!" he screams desperately.*

Wow! Arousal! Wow! He's six, OK, nearly seven. Stay with it—just endure this bit here, this bit of brutal therapy. The mother is now on the other side of the door with a female colleague of mine. She tells me that she had to hold the mother, physically restraining her, because the mother wants to go through the one-way screen, to rescue her dying child, essentially.

Akil's mother displays a clearly unresolved attachment pattern with her son; she is very anxious and over-protective, assisting him as if he were a much younger child, while Akil appears regressive and helpless. Eia Asen's intervention creates an almost shock-like separation between them and links this separation with a demand to Akil. This lets Eia Asen assess both the mother's and Akil's resources in relation to limbic separation and Akil's capacity for self-organising around prefrontal and more age-appropriate demands from an authority figure.

*In the video, Eia Asen enters the room again and says to Akil, who is trying to slip past him and out the door, "It's fine. Your mummy's there, she's going to come back when you've finished. So if you sit down and eat your mummy will come back." Akil tries to slip out the door, but Eia Asen closes*

*it. "Sit down, it's fine, your mummy's there. She's still alive." Akil is bang-*
*ing and clawing at the door, trying to get out. Eia Asen says, "Eat two*
*spoons! Eat two spoons!"*

I'm trying to reassure him, but I'm not trying to calm him down. I
want to see what happens, both in front, in the room, and behind the
screen. And then, of course, I have to do the mopping-up procedure.
I got myself into this dreadful situation, now how do I fix it? Akil is
hyperventilating, but he's still alive, that's a good thing. The mother,
of course, is in a total state of panic. She's breathing much more heav-
ily than him. Earlier, we talked about following, but I'm instructing
him, I'm not following him.

*In the video, Akil rushes over to the table, shoves two spoonfuls into his*
*mouth and yells, "Mummy, mummy, come back. Where are you?" The*
*mother rushes in, kissing and hugging him. Eia Asen says to Akil, "That was*
*quite good. Now eat the rest, or else mummy's going to leave again!"*

Look at that lovely mother. She's so much nicer than me. She wipes
the snot off, she hugs him. At the moment I've got no ambition about
getting her to think about what is going on in this boy, why he's in a
panic, or for the boy to think about why his mother is in that state, for
her to think, etc.—it's not possible at this time.

*In the video, the mother continues to hug Akil, wiping his face, carefully*
*rearranging the dishes on the table, which had been thrown into disarray by*
*the violent commotion, putting everything within easy reach for Akil. Eia*
*Asen says to her, "You don't need to do that. He's a big boy." The mother*
*replies, without conviction, "Yes, he's a big boy." Asen now says firmly to*
*the mother, "Let him eat by himself," and leaves the room. Akil is coughing*
*and sniffling, and the mother asks him, "Why were you crying?"*

The mother goes back to exactly the same over-protective behaviour,
even though I virtually strapped her down in the chair with my
instruction! But at least she stays seated for now.

*In the video, Eia Asen enters the room again and begins to joke with Akil.*
*He listens to his stomach to check if the food is going down properly and*
*announces that "Yes, it is!" To the mother, he says, "Don't plead, he can eat*
*by himself. He can do without that." To Akil he says, "Keep eating, I'll talk*

*to mummy." Akil eats one mouthful after another, while Eia sits behind him, talking to the mother.*

> So I've literally given absolute instructions, I totally managed the context, I totally dominated, I set up a deliberate context.

Here, Eia Asen is drawing on prefrontal structures to establish a separation between Akil and his mother. He has given the mother several clear instructions, but when she is alone in the room with Akil, her habit of over-protection is so strong that she cannot stop herself from helping him or, at least, watching over his every move. Therefore, Eia Asen increases his support for the mother by first engaging in a positive and humorous exchange with Akil, which demonstrates that the boy is handling the situation fine, although he is still somewhat wary of Eia Asen. Next, he frames the generational hierarchy by having a conversation with the mother while Akil is required to keep eating on his own. After talking with the mother for some time, he suggests that she read a book; this is to help her draw her attention back to herself.

*In the video, Eia Asen says to the mother, "You could plead with him, too, you could say, 'Please, my darling, eat!' You could do that." He then says to Akil, who drops his spoon as his attention is caught by this exchange, "Keep eating, keep eating!" The mother says, "I can never leave him alone, he's like a baby. And he says he can't." Eia Asen says to the mother, "Do you believe it?" and she replies, "He tells me I don't love him; if I'm not with him all the time he tells me I don't love him." Asen asks again, "Do you believe that? Has he brainwashed you into believing that? And you fall for it? It's amazing, you fall for that? But do you love him? Yes—so why do you believe it? You're a perfect victim. The reason why I let you in was I was worried about you, I wasn't worried about him, I thought he could cope with it. But the problem was I was really worried about you back there. I thought you were going to crack up, that's why I let you back in, it was not because of him." The mother thinks about this, then looks back to Akil, who is still eating, nervously eyeing Eia Asen. Asen asks her, "If you could look inside his head what do you think you could see? What is he thinking right now about me, you, and so on?" The mother replies, "He's thinking he's not going to come here again." Asen then asks her whether she had brought a book that she might read, so that she had something else to do besides watching over*

*Akil's every move: "Get a novel, if you've got a novel you might be able to finish by the time he's finished his food!"*

Akil eats a little bit more, but she can't help feeding him and helping him. She served three courses at the same time, and she told me, "Because I run a restaurant, I can't help it." And I ask, "What do you do at your restaurant, do you serve them three courses at the same time? Have it all together, eat what you like?" So she has to laugh, and she says, "No, he has to first eat the soup. I cooked it for six hours!!"

In these exchanges, Eia Asen supports the mother's mentalization capacity, first by introducing her to a perspective where her son is strong, while she is fragile, and next by asking her to compare her expectations of her restaurant guests with her expectations of her son.

*In the video, Akil coughs and drops a bit of food, and the mother, startled, reaches out to him. Eia Asen says to the mother, "How difficult is it to lean back?! I'll put a seat belt around you!" The mother now pulls out a book, leans back in her chair and tries to stop focusing on Akil, who keeps watching her, appealing to her. Eia Asen says to the mother, "I'm doing an exam later on to check what you've read." The mother laughs, and Eia Asen leaves the room.*

She may have just pretended to read the book, so I want her to really read it.

*In the video, the mother tries to focus on her book, and Akil is picking at his food but still coughing, choking slightly on the food, dropping the bread and generally trying just about anything to get her attention and to make her feed him.*

So we could say that I now persecute both of them for the next ten or fifteen minutes. But I also connect with the boy in a funny sort of way. He becomes quite interested in what I'm doing, begins to ask me some questions after a little while. He eventually finishes the food. He doesn't want to leave when he's finished. So the mother thinks it's pretty good that it only took him an hour and ten minutes to eat that bit, and since she had paid for two hours of parking, she now wants to discuss the next problem.

*In the video, the mother says, "Maybe we should look at something else I worry about: He can never do his homework. I have to be there continuously,*

*Akil is asking me questions, and it takes two to three hours." During this exchange, Akil is watching both adults carefully. Eia Asen says, "OK, you can do the homework here, but the problem is that I'm not going to be around, I have got other things to do", and then he leaves the room.*

The amazing thing is that this boy does the homework in ten minutes without asking for his mother's help at all. So the mother is totally staggered, "How did that happen!" I say, "Oh, I haven't got a clue, why could it be?" So now I become the mentalizing therapist after being the Germanic therapist, instead of "Do this, do this, do this", I sort of scratch my head and wonder. I become curios, and I say, "Hmm, why could it be that he's doing it, I've got no idea!" The mother has no explanation either, other than probably to think that if he doesn't finish it, the bastard therapist is going to come in again!

*In the video, Eia Asen asks Akil, "Do you want to come back?" With excitement, he says, "Yes, yes, yes!" Eia Asen: "When?" Akil: "Tomorrow?" Eia Asen answers with a smile, "No, it can't be tomorrow."*

So he came back two weeks later with his mother. Again, the family makes up their own context; it's up to them to decide who comes. The mother says her husband works too hard, and he's away on a business trip. This time, we split the session, so that I'm alone with Akil. My female colleague, Natasha, meets with the mother. They watch the video of the previous session, and Natasha asks the mother to think about what she thinks is going on in the boy, and what is going on in herself. Afterwards, Natasha tells me that the mother is very excited while they are doing this.

*In the video, Eia Asen says to Akil, "Your mum wants to talk to my colleague. Do you want to spend a bit of time with me on your own?" Akil, excited and enthusiastic, "Yeah!" They go into the therapy room, and Eia Asen says, "You know, last time you had a real problem being in that room by yourself. And I hear your mum tells me the same thing. Shall we practise being in the room on your own? So, can you do the following things: first, I'm going to sit in the room, and can you go out of the room and see whether I panic like mad when you're out of the room? So I'll be sitting here for about thirty seconds, not more than that, please, and then come back." Akil nods and leaves the room. After thirty seconds he comes back in, and Eia Asen asks, "Do you think I can do it for one minute?" and Akil nods and runs out again. Then they switch, so that Akil stays in the room while Asen leaves.*

*Akil times it, and they keep switching back and forth, all the while increasing the duration, and Akil is growing increasingly confident.*

He manages to spend five minutes in the room on his own, something the mother says has never happened before.

In this brief sequence with Akil, Eia Asen uses both the authoritative direction and the prefrontal capacity for play from the second growth spurt. First, he gives Akil a new, prefrontal perspective on the situation by taking Akil's place as the person who is left behind inside the room and by setting a manageable timeframe. Next, they take turns, building Akil's mastery of this new skill together.

Two weeks later, they come back. This time, both the parents come in with Akil.

*In the video, we see the family entering the room, and Eia Asen says to Akil, "Do you want to sit on your mum's lap, on your dad's lap, on my lap, or on a chair of your own?" Akil replies, "A chair of my own." Now follows a slightly challenging, playful exchange between Eia Asen and Akil. Eia Asen asks, "How old do you have to be to have a chair of your own?" and Akil answers, "Five!" Asen then asks, "And how old do you have to be to sleep on your own?" Akil: "Ten!" Asen: "And how old do you have to be to eat on your own?" Akil answers, with a twinkle in his eye, "Seven!" Eia Asen: "And how old are you now?" Akil: "I'm seven."*

In fact, he's only six. But he's six and eleven months, and he deliberately makes himself older. So that age is significant, I think, as a cue to play with ages, as you will see.

This mutually playful, joking exchange between Eia Asen and Akil creates mental concepts for age-appropriate autonomy and Akil's self-concept in relation to these concepts.

*In the video, Eia Asen says, "And how do you behave as a seven-year-old? Do you think I'm thinking it's a seven-year-old sitting there? Or do you think I think this is a five-year-old sitting there? So what do you think it is about you sitting there that makes me think that you're seven years old?" Akil: "Because I'm being sensible."*

Not an easy question, that, but he *gets* it! This is supposed to be an autistic child with ADHD, just remember that! And as you can see, there's a father sitting there. A very, very nice man, but very, very busy. Genuinely busy, they have a very hard life in London to make their restaurant work, And the mother is also helping out in the restaurant, but the boy is making huge demands on her, so she's not available, and the father needs to work even harder.

*In the video, Eia Asen says to Akil, "I'll ask your mummy and daddy in a while how often you have been sensible since I last saw you. The answer can be never, sometimes, a lot of the time, most of the time, always. What do you think they'll answer?" Akil says, "I think 'sometimes'." The father says, "With me he's sensible a lot of the time." Akil then says to Eia Asen, "And because this morning I kissed daddy, that made him even better." Eia Asen asks, "Because he was kissed?" and Akil says, "Yes." Eia Asen asks, "Daddy sleeps in the morning?" and Akil answers, "Yes, because he comes back at three or four in the morning." Eia Asen then says, "And now I'm going to ask your mum how sensible you've been," and the mother replies, "Sometimes."*

So he read his mum properly. Last time I saw him, in the third session, when I saw him on his own, I interviewed him, as you'll see in a moment. I also gave him a stethoscope. I've got stethoscopes and white coats and things from my past career as a real doctor. And I use them to get the kids to listen to their own thoughts and feelings or to listen to the thoughts and feelings of their parent. I gave Akil a stethoscope and asked him to think about the way he feels anxious and the way he feels sad. I get him to listen to different parts of his body with the stethoscope.

*In the video, Akil is wearing the stethoscope around his neck, and a dialogue ensues as Eia Asen says, "Now, we just practised something, didn't we? What did we practise?" Akil says, "Being in the room for five seconds, ten seconds, twenty seconds . . ." Eia Asen: "And what was that like?" Akil: "Not really scary for me." Eia Asen asks, "Not really. Why wasn't it really scary for you?" Akil answers, "Because I learnt how to not be scared." Eia Asen asks, "And how did you learn that?" Akil: "From my mum." Eia Asen then asks, "How did she teach you that?" and Akil answers, "She said that she'll leave me for . . . if you're scared you won't be clever." Eia Asen asks, "Did she say that? That's good. But sometimes you are scared in your own bedroom, aren't you. What are you scared of?" and Akil answers, "I'm scared of . . . rats. And I'm scared of . . . bats." Eia Asen asks, "Rats and bats. But do you have that come into your bedroom? Have you ever seen any in your bed?" Akil says, "No, but once I've seen a mice." and Eia Asen says, "And do you think . . . What do the mice do, eat you up?" Akil laughs and says, "Noooo! They just come to you. But I am more scared of . . . And I'm also scared of mosquitoes. And bees." Eia Asen asks, "But do they come into your bedroom? Why are you scared of—they could come into this room now, couldn't they, what would you do?" Akil: "I would just run away." Eia Asen asks, "And in the bedroom?" Akil answers, "Hmmm . . . put some fly spray." Asen continues, "So tell me one more thing about your mummy and your daddy. Who helps you more not to be scared? Your mummy or your daddy?" Akil answers, "My daddy." Asen: "How come?" Akil: "Because when I'm sometimes scared he always comes to me." Eia Asen says, "And your mum doesn't do that." Akil answers, "Sometimes she does."*

So he's able to differentiate between the anxiety-containing abilities of father *vs.* mother.

In this sequence, Eia Asen asks reality-testing questions and explores Akil's capacity for building representations of executive agency, both of which are key coping skills in the second growth spurt.

*In the video, Eia Asen says, "So if you shout and scream, your dad comes?" and Akil answers, "Yes. But I don't shout and scream." With a smile, Eia Asen says, "You don't, no. And at what point, do you think, should you sleep on your own? How old would you have to be to sleep on your own?" Akil answers, "Seven . . . Eleven."*

He's going up!

*In the video, Eia Asen says, "Eleven? Seven? You're seven soon, aren't you?" Akil (insistent): "I'm seven!" Eia Asen, with a smile, "Errrrhh— you're seven, when?" Akil answers, "I'm been seven," and Eia Asen answers with playful scepticism, "Is that true? Look into my face, and tell me if that's true." Akil looks at him innocently and says, "Yes," and Eia Asen replies, "Now, look at your face . . ."*

I've got a camera, it's a very simple one, and you can put the viewfinder over, so he can see himself in that viewfinder. So he looks at himself now, as we speak.

*In the video, Eia Asen says, "What does that face tell you?" Akil answers, still with an innocent look on his face, "I'm seven," and Asen says, "If you saw a face like that, would you believe that person, or would you think that he was telling some porky? Do you think there is something in that face that made one think, 'Oh, maybe he's not telling the truth totally'?" Akil answers, still with an innocent air, "I think that person is telling the truth." Asen then says, "How would you know if he was not telling the truth? If he was only six years and quite a few months but not quite seven yet, how you know that he was not telling you the truth? What would that face look like?"*

There is widespread laughter in the audience. Eia Asen shakes his head: "He's running rings around me . . . So I go on a bit about this to see if he can change his view. I don't manage particularly well . . ."

*In the video, Akil says, "I'm nearly seven, but I lapse sometimes." Eia Asen asks, "Do you behave like a seven-year-old most of the time?" and Akil answers, "Sometimes, but yesterday I behaved like ten-year-old." Eia Asen asks, with curiosity, "Really, what were you doing?" Akil explains, "There was a man and a lady who bought me a violin, and they're going to buy me a drum. A drum-kit to play on. And we were being so kind to them, they even said 'we will buy an extra one.' And the lady has a violin, and it's electric." Eia Asen then asks, "Now look at that face now. When you look at that face, did the person who told the story tell the truth?" and Akil answers, "Yes." Eia Asen asks, "And the person who talked about the birthday before, do you think he told just the truth or only some of the truth?" Akil answers, "The truth." Eia Asen: "Totally the truth?" Akil, with a smile playing in his otherwise innocent expression: "Yes."*

There is more laughter in the audience. Eia Asen says, "OK. I should give up here but I couldn't quite do it . . . I'll just fast-forward here."

*In the video, Eia Asen asks Akil, "What's the date today?" Akil says, "April the 5th," and Eia Asen replies, "Gosh, you know a lot. So is April the 5th before or after May the 19th?" [Akil's birthday] and Akil answers triumphantly, "It's after!"*

Laughter in the audience. Eia Asen comments, "He's outfoxed me, as you have already seen!"

Throughout this exchange, Eia Asen and Akil play with their internal representations of each other's internal representations. Akil is well aware that he is tricking Asen, and that Asen is aware of this and allows it to happen, plays with it, and tries to challenge Akil to tell the truth, in part by checking if he is actually able to keep a straight face when he looks at himself in the camera monitor. Akil wins this playful joust in words, with warm acceptance from Eia Asen. On the prefrontal level, this demonstrates the same principle that we saw in both Peter Levine's and Jukka Mäkelä's work, where the powerful adult imposes a "handicap" on himself to let the child win.

*In the video, Eia Asen says to Akil, "And do you sometimes behave like a two-year-old?" Akil replies, "No!" Asen asks, "Do you remember when I first saw you?" Akil says, "Yes. I behaved like a one-year-old!" Throughout this conversation Akil was clearly relaxed and happy, spinning playfully on the office chair.*

So here you've got fantastic self-appreciation. He behaved like a one-year-old. And he talks then about the eating and all that kind of stuff.

*In the video, Eia Asen says to Akil, "A one-year-old. I got it wrong, OK. So what was it you were doing then that would have made me think that you were one year old?" Akil says, "Didn't listen, of course." Eia Asen: "Didn't listen. Something else?"*

*Akil: "Didn't eat." Eia Asen asks, "Yeah. But you did eat, but how did you eat?"*

*Akil replies, "My mum feeding me..." (sputtering, giggling).*

So—just a bit of audience interaction: how many of you think this child has got a severe autistic disorder? [Laughter.] OK. What about ADHD? OK. So this makes me feel quite positive about the boy, I must say. But the question is, can the parents see it that way as well? So I said to the boy, "If I show this tape to your mum and dad, what do you think they would think? Would it be a good thing, a bad thing, an embarrassment?" And he says, "No, I want them to see what I say to you."

So now we are watching on a laptop in session number four. And I'm interested in the parents' responses. And the technique I would use is

I would stop the recording and say, "So why do you think he's saying that, and why's he doing that?" And "What do you think your mum and dad are thinking about this," and so on. So, as we watch this on a laptop, I'm using the mentalizing frame and getting them to understand why he was saying that or the other.

And when both parents and Akil see situations like that, this beautiful contact between mother and son, one option would be to look at the mother–son dyad and how that might exclude the father. For example, we might say, "Oh, what a beautiful couple, they're so beautiful, those two", and then ask the father, "How are you feeling when you see that, Mr Maher?" That would be a way of raising the temperature again. But I decide not to do it. I decide to stay with those moments of Akil's huge competence, fantastic sense of humour, his ability to look at himself, also from a distance or from a humorous distance. The self-assessment. Only two or three weeks ago, when he probably hated my guts and he couldn't eat and so on . . . To put him into the right age range, he *is* actually like one-year-old in that scene, he's not like a two-year-old, he's quite right.

Using video feedback, to look at yourself from the outside, it's not a specific technique, but it's something that I think we use more and more in our work, to good effect. For example, the father also wanted to see the recording from the first session where Akil refused to eat. And what's fascinating is that the mother sits there and watches it, and she is almost in the same state watching the video as she was when being out of the room four weeks earlier. Very tense, full of anxiety. And Akil—he is relaxed, laughing. And the dad is very respectful, he doesn't laugh, but you can see the . . .

So it makes me think that there is some work that one needs to do, probably with the mother, or with the mother and father. And that's the next step of the work that we do. And, in fact, because I'm often a bit busier than my colleague, she decides to do this, so we are now in sessions five and six, two-week intervals, and the mother is seen on her own. This is the context that we've built with them, because at the end of the last session, I said to each of them, "We can meet again. Who do you think should meet? What would be the advantages of all of you coming? What would be the advantages and disadvantages of only two of you coming, one of you coming, father and mother and so on." And the mother said, "When I saw this tape again, when I remember this situation, I know there's something inside me that I need to think about or work with." So, she had two sessions on her own, and she talked about the horrendous circumstances around the birth, how the child almost died, how in her mind the child that she sees—this lovely boy—is the child that she remembers was almost dying. So she sees him as sort of mortally ill, a child that needs to be fed, fed, fed, and fed, and so on. So, my colleague does some work on that; two sessions with the mother. Again, we haven't got a luxurious service where we could offer substantially more, but these sessions, I can tell you, were not ten minutes, they were one hour long each of them, which is rare. So, the mother was given some help, and, of course, part of that work is to think about how her son, Akil, constructs himself as a result of her view of him. So she sees him, treats him in a particular way, and that has an effect on his view of himself, which is a difficult clinical issue to deal with.

The mother managed to loosen her anxious focus on her son enough that she was able to focus on herself and her own needs, which helped her realise that she needed to address her horrifying and unresolved image of dying infant to be able to see her actual, current son as the big, healthy boy that he has become. This ability to distinguish the past from the present and to allow the new perspective to change the self-narrative and the representation of the other is another essential element in the development of mentalization during the second growth spurt.

> So, here we are, a few months later. Akil is doing well in school, he has friends, he eats properly, he is doing generally well in all contexts, he sleeps on his own . . . *but* he is still a total mother's mind-reader type of person, continuously fixed on her mind, as if the only way he can construct himself is through the mind of his mother. In the next clip you will see how he always checks with his mother before he says anything. It's like a magnet being pulled. The mother has got a very expressive face. She's a very warm, caring person.

> *In the video, Eia Asen asks Akil, "What's mum going to say about the eating, 'good' and so on?" The boy looks to his mother. Eia Asen points out that Akil does this, and the mother tries to hide her face to prevent Akil from "reading" her. Asen says to Akil, "Can you see what mum is trying to do; she's trying to hide."*

> She's probably worried about being told off by the German doctor! [Eia Asen is German-born and repeatedly joked about his "harsh, Germanic" style] Or maybe she's got it herself, without even thinking about me.

*In the video, Eia Asen says to Akil, "Maybe we should put a mask on her head, what do you think?" Akil was up for trying that.*

My thinking is, of course, that he's so good at mind-reading, but what about his own mind, how much can he have his own space, his own thinking, and so on? Or can he only construct his own inner world through the mother? Now, the mother thinks that the child is normal, but the paediatrician who made the diagnosis has written to her that she needs to come in for a follow-up appointment—this is six months later—because "your child has very severe autism". So the medical system is reinforcing the autism idea. My way is just the moralistic approach, just like Haldor: "Forget these idiots," although I don't say it quite like that . . . Instead, I say to the mother, "I don't think an autistic child would be as good as him, I don't think he's autistic. They cannot read minds like that, let me tell you: They cannot."

*In the video, the mother puts on a mask. She picks it at random, with her eyes closed, so she does not know what the mask looks like, that is, what the boy sees. In her first attempt to put it on, she turns the mask upside down, so the hole for the mouth is in her forehead, and they all laugh. She then manages to turn it right side up. Eia Asen says to Akil, "What do you think she is feeling right now? Look at her, because I know you're always looking at her." Akil leans over, gets up close, tries to "read" her despite the mask.*

So, we can use masks in many different ways. Here, we ask the mother to pick a mask without knowing what that mask is. She picks out a mask at random, puts the mask on but does not know what her son sees when he sees her. It's different when the mother knows it's a pig's mask. When she knows she looks like a pig to him, then maybe she constructs what he says in relation to knowing what she looks like at that moment. But when she doesn't know it, it becomes even more interesting and sophisticated for her to guess what the boy sees now in her.

After this session they were part of a group, which they met with twice, and that helped them to get some feedback from the other families, as I described earlier. There have been a few sessions since then, and the session I want to show you is where they've got to now. And that session starts in an interesting way—I hadn't seen them for a while. The parents come with the boy, and it so happens that there is a globe of the world in a corner of that room.

*In the video, Akil goes over to the globe and examines it, and Eia Asen stops his interaction with the parents and follows him as the parents watch attentively. Eia Asen says to Akil, "Where are we now? Put the globe on the table."*

I follow him for once! So, one thing that hasn't been explored, but which is very often a big issue with the families we see, is their migration history, the trauma they suffered, and so on, and to what extent this is part of a family narrative in which the child can also be included.

*Eia Asen says to Akil, "Tell me where your dad is from." Akil points to Iraq on the globe. "Yes. And where is mum from?" Akil points. Eia Asen says, "Yes. And where did your parents live before they came here?" and Akil replies, "My mum lived in Bulgaria before she came here. And dad . . . in Iraq." Eia Asen says, "Iraq. And . . . I heard something about Turkey at some point?" and the mother says, "Yes. Before we came here, your mother lived in Turkey. And your father the same." The father adds, "Your mother was born in Bulgaria, and your father was born in Iraq," and the mother continues, "We lived in Turkey for some time." Eia Asen asks Akil, "And have they explained to you why that is?" Akil looks slightly puzzled at Asen, who tells him, "Here we've got people who are terribly good at research. You want to tell them about research? Do you know what research is—it's a nosy little boy asking 'Why did you end up in Turkey?'"*

So, this is something that is often very important for the migration families that we deal with; that story, and what parts of that story can be shared.

And there's a very sad mother story, there's a lot of sadness, the father's life in Iraq; the mother's family lived in Bulgaria, they were persecuted there, because they are ethnic Turks, and so on.

Another thing that the mother said to us the last time, about two months ago, is, "You know something: I'm ready now to have another baby." They've talked to the boy about having a baby, so this is another theme that comes up, and it's amazing how the boy talks about another baby, and what kind of baby he wants: "I hope I get the right thing."

*In the video, Eia Asen says to Akil: "Are you nine now?" Akil is quick to answer "Eight."*

There you are, he's learnt something! All these trick questions! So, I look at the role of the father in the household. The typical stuff you do: when he's there, when he's not there, the difference and so on. How does he keep up? I get the mother's story, the father's story. We now hear about the grandmother. The grandparents are moving in from Turkey, and she's talking about how the grandmother is there at the moment, and the grandmother is undoing everything that the mother does. She feels that grandmother remembers how babyish and how ill Akil was, and how his life was threatened when he was so young, and the grandmother was present then, and she is still traumatised by it. Now, the grandmother has moved in with them for a few months, and she infantilises or babies Akil. So that's work we have to do, and in two weeks' time, we're doing home-base work with the grandmother there.

In the next clip, the mother and I are talking about another theme: there is space in the family for another child, but can Akil share this space with another child? The mother's sister has a daughter who is four or five years old, and she is a bit like a sister to Akil when she visits. Akil's mother explains that after spending time with the girl, Akil doesn't want to see any more of her, he doesn't want to involve the girl in anything, and the mother wishes that he would.

*In the video, Eia Asen asks, "She's an only child, is she?" and the mother says, "He is an only child, and she is an only child." Asen then asks, "But are you saying he would find it difficult to share his time with a baby?" Akil's mother says, "Yes, and he was complaining . . ." Asen ask the mother, "Has he put an order in [for the kind of baby he wants]?" He then turns to Akil and asks, "So do you think it's a bad idea if mum and dad had another baby?" and Akil says, "Nah." Eia Asen insists, "I would like to hear it from you . . .?" Akil replies, "The sort of thing I want is a big . . . a quiet baby who does not disturb everything and . . ." he then goes on to complain about his cousin, who acts like a baby, interrupts, and demands attention constantly.*

He wants a well-behaved baby! Well, you can't order them, not even on the Internet!

*Eia Asen says to Akil, "So you say that if there's a baby in the family, it has to be a well-behaved one?" Akil: "Yeah." Eia Asen teases him a little: "Like you?" Akil laughs a little and says, "When I was five years old, I was not very well-behaved."*

So he remembers that he wasn't very well-behaved at some point.

*Akil complains that his cousin wants the same thing every single day, "Because she watches* Happy Feet *every single day!"*

The stupid girl, it's the worst, *Happy Feet,* every day! Boring, right, boring, boring, boring! So, I ask him for tips [on how to deal with poorly behaved children]. He's got many, many good tips. But I'm not going show you the tips, because I want to show you something else.

You may remember, when I spoke to Akil on camera, he said, "Yesterday I behaved like ten," because there were these nice, kind people with a violin? And, in fact, one of these people gave him a violin; they also had an electric violin, perhaps for the future. Last Friday, he came straight from his first violin exam. After just one year he plays really quite nicely, you'll hear him play in a minute. So, he's brought the violin, he wants to play for us. And you'll see what I do with that in terms of rhythm.

*In the video, Akil plays his violin—his mother offers to hold the sheet music. Eia Asen asks the mother, "Are you a music stand, or are you a mother?!"*

A lot of work to be done there! Why shouldn't mum be a music stand, I'm being a bit harsh, aren't I?

*Akil plays the violin for a while. Then Eia Asen plays a short piece on his violin while Akil listens.*

He's asked me whether I've got an electric violin, which I have. So I brought it in for that session, last week, to have a bit of fun, basically.

*Akil and Eia Asen jam on their violins. It gets pretty intense. At one point, Akil objects: "No! You can't it play it like eeeeee [drawn-out, sliding tone]"*

But I like schmaltzing, you know!

*Eia Asen says to Akil, "I'm going to play something for you, and you have to tell me, what do you think is the mood, or what's the story behind it?" He plays a short passage and asks who the person in the music might be.*

*Akil answers, "Sleeping Beauty!" Eia Asen then asks, "Sleeping Beauty. Is that person very happy or . . .?" and Akil answers, "Very sad." Eia Asen then asks, "Why is that?" and Akil answers, "Because the music is very sad."*

> So I get into a dialogue with him, playing different kinds of music to see whether he can pick up the musical state that's behind it. And we end up . . . no, that's too embarrassing, I don't want to show it, but I play a Bulgarian folk song for the mother. But that's too schmaltzy!

By asking Akil to imagine the person portrayed in the music, Eia Asen is asking Akil to use his mentalization capacity on quite a high level, since he has to be able to recognise and symbolise the limbic feeling in a piece of music and relate it to a story, which he does without any difficulty.

> That's where we are at the moment. And for the boy, it was very important to show his skills . . . probably for me as well . . . This boy, if we wind the clock back a year, he felt totally persecuted by me, he's come, he's doing extremely well in his life. We still have to do some work with his mum and mum's mum, and also a bit with the father. But the difficulties at school have gone; he's got a huge friendship network. For the mother, it's taken about a year to see him as a normal boy, while it was easier for the father. The fact that they're thinking about having another baby, of course, is a marvellous way forward. In the last session, Akil said to me, "I'm worried about what may happen to mummy when the new baby comes, because we've been told the story in school where the mummy dies when the baby is born." So there is that story also in the background.

## Summary

This chapter described the second wave of development in higher-order mental competences and reviewed a therapy process that challenged the prefrontal compass and the capacities that emerge in the second wave of development. A characteristic of this process was Akil's unresolved attachment pattern with his mother. By challenging Akil on an age-appropriate level and with the use of humour, Eia Asen was able to work with Akil's capacities in a mentalizing process. The process also addressed the mother's unresolved attachment with

Akil, which appeared very fixated and required individual work with the mother, separate from the therapy with Akil. In relation to both Akil and his mother, Eia Asen used mentalizing narratives and reality testing. Eia Asen's approach was confrontational, but, thanks to a consistently humorous and light-hearted approach, he managed to make Akil and his mother see themselves from an outside perspective and engage in a mentalizing process. This challenged the higher level of mentalization that both Akil and his mother now had access to. Thus, Eia Asen operated in the zone of proximal development with both Akil and his mother.

CHAPTER SEVEN

# The therapist in the role of caravan leader

"The only way for a child to feel truly safe is to have someone show the way. And when the child feels safe there is room for exploration, joy and having fun"

(Jukka Mäkelä)

Psychotherapy with children relies on an experience of under-standing and reacting physically and mentally to the child's state by experiencing the child through eye contact, the body, prosody (the rhythm, register, and emotional tone of the voice) etc. The expanded intersubjective space that matures in the normally developing child seven to nine months after birth leads to new oppor-tunities and new ways of being with others. Experiences are shared as they occur, and the way of being with others unfolds in the moment, before the experience is conveyed or rephrased in words. Change is based on lived experiences, and the nervous system develops through subjective experiences as they unfold. As pointed out by Stern (2004), events must be *lived*, with feelings and actions taking place in real time, in the real world, with real people. Stern mentions three mental states that are essential for early intersubjective relatedness. One is the ability to engage in a field of joint attention, the second is the experience of having shared intentions, and the third is to be able to take part in other people's affective states, all of which are conditions for a therapeutic process.

The therapeutic process is largely about the therapist's ability to create the sense of being mentally present with the child and to listen to the child's signals but also to take responsibility for change processes. In this chapter, we look at this asymmetrical responsibility in relation to generating sustained change processes, as the therapist, just like the affectively attuned mother, initiates the self-regulating and identity-building process.

## The importance of the therapist's authenticity, grounding, and full presence

As mentioned in Chapter One, change processes in psychotherapy occur when two people enter into an intersubjective contact in a present moment. This involves a feeling of "I know that you know that I know", or "I feel that you feel that I feel" (Stern, 2004, p. 75) and implies the ability to grasp another person's emotions. In the absence of an intersubjective connection, a meeting often produces a level of anxiety that mobilises defensive strategies. The point is not to satisfy the child's needs, but to understand the child and engage in a shared experience.

The experience of being met and accepted without judgment affirms the child's experience of the world. This form of recognition implies an immediate emotional presence, accessibility and self-delimitation. The moment is always new, yet the relational behaviour patterns are repeated, without ever being quite the same. In the here-and-now situation, something is unfolding that has never unfolded in quite the same way before, and each moment contains a possibility of embracing the new along with aspects of previous experiences. Experiences of reciprocity arise in the improvisational process in the moment when the process unfolds, and these experiences contain both participants' previous internal representations. In the intersubjective field, the range of possible experiences expands when the experiences become accessible and have room to unfold. We attune with each other's affects and share them whenever possible, and we connect by meeting on the same level of intensity and with matching emotions.

Hafstad and Øvreeide (in Hart, 2011) emphasise the innate human potential to engage in rhythmic and mutually attuned interactions with others, as we express ourselves and our inner states and experience others doing the same. The child is vitalised when he or she is met by a marked vocal prosody and rhythm from adults. When adults show that they share the child's states, emotions, and needs the child responds, and the failure to receive this form of synchronisation in childhood will result in developmental problems. As Øvreeide points out, "sharing the mental state of the moment becomes the critical point in this kind of essential support . . . We become present in each other's states and needs. 'The other's' state becomes 'our own'" (Øvreeide, 2001, p. 25). By actively tuning into the child, the therapist becomes visible to the child. Thus, the child becomes aware of both the therapist and of his or her own states—in the compass model we call this an ego-altercentric participation in the limbic compass. A key aspect of the developmental process is, thus, to see oneself through someone else's eyes, which is what happens in mutually experienced present moments. Through the therapist's curiosity and attunement, the child's internal representations enter into an intersubjective space with the therapist that is different from the intersubjective field where the internal representations originated. It is within this intersubjective field that the transformation of the child's experiential world occurs; it is the potential for experiences that contains the transformative potential.

At its core, empathy rests on the ability to match the other's affect and to respond with resonance. Positive attunement builds trust and acts as the driving force in establishing attachment bonds. The therapist needs to create a vitalising positive attunement with the child in order to use this background of resonance and synchronicity to form attachment bonds with the child that will support a development and a dampening of previous relational strategies that have been hampering psychological development. When the therapist is empathically attuned with child's internal state, the contact is enhanced and vitalised (Stern, 1984; Trevarthen, 1979).

The present moments lead to an emotional vulnerability that might produce an experience of self-exposure. It is important for the therapist to be comfortably grounded in his own personality and not, for example, to be frightened and withdraw, but remain emotionally present and accessible to the child. The emotional accessibility helps to create a sense of calm. In the relationship with asymmetrical responsibility, the therapist has to distinguish between affects that belong to the child and those that belong to him/herself and be able to contain the child's emotions without merging with them (Morgan, 1998; Schibbye, 2005). The psychotherapist's emotional involvement and sense of confidence in the precise timing of his or her own sensations are crucial. The traumatisation that occurs in solitude needs to be healed through contact.

At the conference, Haldor Øvreeide pointed out that, in a dialogical process that deals with difficult, emotionally challenging subjects, the child will often not be prepared to engage with the topic and stay with it. When the therapist addresses the incident or the challenge, we can expect the child to take another initiative. The therapist establishes an initial contact and may expect the child to follow, but once the therapist addresses the challenging issue the child might break off by introducing a different initiative, as we saw in the video clip with Olaf, where he says, "I want to draw a sunflower." In the example, Haldor chose to follow Olaf's initiative, which enabled him to proceed with a new initiative. The therapist should expect to move towards and then away from the key issue: in order to maintain contact with emotionally challenging issues, Olaf has to feel that he has control of the process. That is not necessarily because the issues or topics are too challenging; the key is the relationships, not the topics *per se*. It is, therefore, crucial for Haldor to support Olaf's self-regulation by following his initiative. This gives Olaf the experience that "I am able to control the process myself; the adult is not in complete control of the process." The key is to allow the child to move in and out of the dialogue.

In the therapy process, the therapist needs to strike the right balance between attachment and autonomy and between mutual regulation and self-regulation. Some children who have grown up in insecure attachment patterns will have retreated into their own inner world, isolating themselves as a form of self-protection. When the therapist respects this need for psychological or physical detachment, the child feels understood. The detachment is used to organise, reorganise, and control the arousal level in order to achieve emotional balance and be able to organise on a cognitive level: self-regulation functions. This withdrawal reflects a psychobiological need and supports the development of coping strategies. Infants may achieve detachment by avoiding eye contact, blocking their ears or closing their eyes.

Many children convey a superficial message of wanting to be left alone. It would be a mistake, however, to take this message at face value: being left alone or abandoned is also something that terrifies children. To be found despite their withdrawal or avoidant behaviour, these children need an empathic invitation that seeks to include them in a pleasant relationship—a relationship where they feel that they are truly being seen. The child needs to be the focus of adult attention in an intense, personal way in order to feel a connection. The goal is to make sure that the child feels that he or she is "seen" and "heard". Engaging activities include pleasant stimulation, variation as well as a new perspective on life that enables the child to understand that surprises can be fun, and that new experiences can be pleasant. Activities that promote engagement usually involve eye contact, possibly physical contact, play, fun, attention to the other's reactions, and, in many cases, moments of shared surprise and pleasure (Hart, 2011).

## *The responsibility always rests with the person at the top of the hierarchy*

No one can learn to understand the feelings of another human being without having a shared bond that is created in the improvisational process and the present moments. Even small non-verbal attitudes, for example, the way in which the therapist looks at the child, can produce positive relational experiences, and in the therapeutic process it is possible to establish a relationship that is different from a possibly insecure attachment that might be part of the child's background, based on previous relationships. The development of an affective and mentalizing capacity is only possible in a close relationship with a significant other (Fonagy, 1999).

In the carer–child relationship, the carer supports the child in engaging in a social context where he or she encounters learning opportunities. Also in that relationship, the child "borrows" the mother's more highly developed consciousness to use as "scaffolding"

(Bruner, 1985). The child expresses his or her needs, and the carer responds and takes responsibility. In any asymmetrical relationship, including that of mother–child, teacher–student, therapist–client, there is an uneven distribution of responsibility. Like the carer, the psychotherapist has to take responsibility for his or her objectives and be aware of the asymmetrical relationship. As in the child–carer relationship, the optimal development of the therapeutic relationship depends on an equal and equally engaged relationship between the therapist and the child, but this is framed by an asymmetrical distribution of responsibility where the therapist takes responsibility for the setting, attunement, and navigation. The therapist has to provide a space for the child's self-organisation and meet the child within his or her zone of proximal development (Øvreeide, 2001).

An underlying condition for emotional attunement is that two individuals have a shared focus. This forms a preverbal and nonverbal dialogue and a complicated piece of human choreography. All good therapy, regardless of format, is supportive. Winnicott (1960) has used the term "holding", and Bion (1962) the term "containing function" to describe this supportive aspect, which is an indispensable condition of any psychological development. In many respects, these terms are similar to Fonagy's term "marked mirroring" (cf. Hart & Schwartz, 2008). "Holding" and "containing" are key aspects of the therapy process, since the carer has probably not been able to contain the child's feelings sufficiently; thus, these experiences have not been attuned with the child in a manner that enabled integration.

The child brings those personality patterns that have developed, whatever they might be, into the therapy. Winnicott (1971) underlined that the therapist must have an intuitive understanding of the child's emotional history and level of development as well as a theory about the child's emotional development and an understanding of the relationship between the child and his or her environment. A child who grew up in an environment with insensitive or chaotic carers will often meet his or her surroundings with distrust and lack confidence. The lack of positive childhood experiences can lead to a fundamental distrust of the therapist. A predictable emotional environment, in which the therapist consistently expresses "containment" through marked mirroring can then become an important part of the therapeutic process, where the child develops a trusting relationship with the therapist.

In the therapy process, the therapist is curious about the child's mental images of the world, and the child knows that he or she shares this world with the therapist. In order to share an experience with the child, the therapist has to be authentic, meaning that the therapist's body language, emotional expressions, verbal expressions, and internal experience need to be internally coherent and in correspondence with the interaction. Correspondence between the internal and external world is a key aspect of authenticity. The child should be able to approach the therapist without fear of being invaded and without feeling separation and abandonment. In therapy, it is important to create patterns not only for being with another, but, specifically, for being with another in the face of mutual differences. Improvisation in therapy makes the process unpredictable, and change is achieved by modifying the framework to a degree that the child is able to handle. When the framework is reorganised, the child experiences stressful moments, and the process might best be described as a series of minor crises.

In the parent–infant relationship, the role of the parents involves taking responsibility for the safety of the young child. Children require physical regulation, and, as part of their development during the first year of life, they also require emotional regulation. This co-regulation of the child is a key part of being a parent. The parents initiate interactions, organise and regulate the child's experiences, set boundaries, and provide direction and guidance. It is crucial for the child's sense of security to know that there is someone around who is more capable than the child. The adult conveys the message that "You are safe here, with me, because I know how to take care of you." Children need an inner sense that there is, in Bowlby's (1988) words, someone who is "bigger, stronger, wiser and kind" who takes charge. Without this structure in place, most of the child's energy is aimed at preparing for the unpredictable and at trying to control the immediate environment, especially the people who populate this environment. If the persons in the child's immediate world are too scary, the child learns to control every aspect of his or her own behaviour in order to follow the adult's every whim. One might say that in a healthy relationship, the parents lend the child their own internal organisation—metaphorically, they act as the child's prefrontal cortex (see Chapter Five).

## The role as caravan leader

A frightened, chaotic, and unhappy child needs firm, confident, and playful leadership to be drawn into the interaction with the therapist. The therapist should initiate interactions and include the child in the activity without waiting for the child to "choose" to engage in a relationship. To imitate the process of co-regulation with the parents, the therapist has to maintain a rhythmic and sequential process with a beginning, a middle, and an end. Many of the things that happen in Theraplay, for example, are about using parts of the body, counting fingers and toes and commenting on muscles, smiles, etc. At the conference, the concept of the therapist as the secure "caravan leader" was brought up several times. Jukka Mäkelä pointed out the importance of the therapist taking the lead, because the therapy involves doing things that are "dangerous"; for example, being physically close and engaging in intense contact with the child. Handling this contact can be scary for a child, so the therapist has to do something to let the child know that there is another world—a world that lies outside the child's previous field of experience. By being intensely attentive to the child, the therapist expresses an interest: "Who are you? I need you to tell me who you are, and how I can support you." The therapist seeks eye contact because this is a uniquely human act. Human eyes are more demonstrative than the eyes of any other species, because the white of the eye makes very visible who is looking at whom. Humans also have a large number of tiny facial muscles that make the area around the eyes very expressive. It is crucial that the therapist never requires a child to look him or her in the eye; however, when eye contact is made, it should be treated as very meaningful. In Theraplay, Jukka Mäkelä explained, it is also important to talk about the child's unique characteristics: the therapist comments on whether the child is a boy or a girl, the colour of the child's eyes, skin colour, hair colour, how strong and beautiful the child is, any special marks, etc. The therapist notices little injuries and deals with scratches and cuts, which is normally a basic aspect of attachment behaviour. The first time the parents of a newborn child look at their child, they typically notice these features—whether it is a boy or a girl, and whether the child has five fingers and five toes on each hand and foot. That is how a Theraplay course often begins, and even 15–16-year-olds, surprisingly, are still interested in having someone notice how many fingers and toes they have.

Jukka Mäkelä also pointed out that in the asymmetrical relationship it is important to make sure that the child is successful in the activities the therapist suggests. The therapist designs the activities to make sure that the child cannot fail. This involves setting the bar low enough and also simply initiating an activity and seeing whether the child comes along. If the child does not follow, or keep up, there is no failure involved, since no demands were made. If the child does keep up, the therapist can say, "Wow, you're really good at that," which means that the child is guaranteed success. This creates a system where the child is affirmed as being good at the things he or she needs to master, and it creates a setting where the child can experience mastery and accomplishment in contact with another person. When misattunement occurs in therapy, the therapist always takes the responsibility and supports the child in the experience.

Eia Asen pointed to the importance in child therapy of building a strong connection with the children where they feel *validated* as strong individuals and non-fragile beings. This feeling of being validated will lay the groundwork for a new self-concept. If the parents witness the validation, that will help them support the child.

Haldor Øvreeide said that *dependence* is a very important part of the child's conditions and development potential. The child needs to be able to express him/herself and act adaptively by following a *bigger* person. Jukka Mäkelä expanded on this thought by adding that the child needs this bigger person, both for security and as a source of relevant information about life. In that sense, the behaviour of this bigger person plays a very important role for the child's development. In a way, the child is always in a problematic power position because the bigger person is free to pick and choose, and it is crucial that this person makes choices that are appropriate in relation to the child's needs and developmental states. Thus, the power aspect of the relationship, especially in relation to parents or carers, is a key issue to consider.

### Structure and predictability

Jukka Mäkelä has previously described (Hart, 2011) that children need predictability and, therefore, seek confirmation of internal representations, even when these representations are maladaptive. Due to the plasticity of the brain, neural patterns may change when the child encounters variations and changes in the interaction patterns that he or she expects from others. Relational development work consists in finding ways to communicate with the child that can change his or her internal representations and provide the necessary developmental support. The child needs support in relation to his or her current stage of personality development. This means that the child needs support in the areas where he or she seeks competence and mastery and needs to be given opportunities to demonstrate independence in the areas where he or she has already achieved mastery.

Therapy needs to create a setting that is well-structured, clear, unambiguous, manageable, and predictable—in other words, it needs to provide a macro-regulatory framework, a virtual "frontal lobe corset", that prepares the child for what is going to happen. The frontal lobe corset consists of structure/framing, rhythms, predictability, preparation, and the ability to feel with the child without feeling like the child. An insecure child with a fragile nervous system that easily disintegrates is best able to live out his or her potential when the therapist creates a safe and secure situation that provides space for containing the child's insecurities and creates a setting characterised by relevant demands.

The therapy itself also needs to be structured. Structure involves such factors as having a regular seat close to the child and having materials that are introduced in a structured approach, which is pre-planned based on a prior assessment of the particular areas where the child needs developmental support. After making a plan, the therapist also needs to look at the child, listen to what the child has to say, and notice the child's special way of being, which might make it necessary to modify the plan and do something else that meets the child's needs on the given day. The point is to remain receptive and attuned to the child's reactions to the activities and to guide the child through a series of interactive experiences that revolve around regulation, organisation, and security.

When adults take responsibility for the structure, the child is relieved of the burden of deciding the next step or exercising control and securing his or her own safety. Children with emotional or behavioural problems generally have a difficult time with control aspects and sometimes try to take control and manage events that exceed their developmental capacity. For children to develop adaptive autonomy and independence, adults need to provide leadership. This is especially important if the children have had disorganised parents who were unable to manage their own lives, or if the child was born with challenges that make it difficult to establish structure. Theraplay, for example, puts a clear emphasis on providing structure for all children, but especially for children who are hyperactive and dys-regulated and for children who self-regulate too much and who are self-confident and controlling. On the other hand, the structure should be loosened when a child is perfectionist, timid, or rigid. Simply stick-ing to the rules and telling these children not to do anything until they are told could intensify their rigidity. The therapist still has a plan, but deliberately chooses to take a slightly less structured approach. In these cases, the structure may simply involve talking about what is going to happen, what is happening now, and what just happened.

Structure makes it safe to pursue the spontaneous interest that builds the personality structure. Jukka Mäkelä sometimes mentions the Arabic proverb, "The dogs bark, but the caravan goes on". The caravan leader has to know the way and make sure that everyone arrives safely at the next oasis before nightfall. The dogs are free to chase lizards and other exciting things along the trail, but the caravan cannot stop every single time, as it would risk being swallowed up by the desert. In all good child therapy, the therapist assumes the role of caravan leader. Fortunately, there are many oases on the therapy trail, and they are not far apart, so there is plenty of time to follow the spontaneous ideas of a playful child. Nevertheless, the fundamental principle remains the same: the only way for a child to feel truly safe is to have someone show the way. When the child feels safe, there is room for exploration, joy, and having fun.

Structure is, thus, a condition for releasing the potential of a child's spontaneity and creative energy. In Theraplay, for example, the struc-ture derives from the therapist's stance of being simultaneously strong and receptive, well-prepared and in control, constantly open to the child's signals, but also ready to show the child new possibilities that might otherwise have gone unnoticed. To a certain extent, the thera-pist must provide both predictability and surprises. To achieve this, the therapist has to pre-plan the session and map out the activities to be able to lead the caravan to the next oasis, even if the trail temp-orarily becomes unclear. The therapist uses simple statements instead of questions to invite the child to move along.

Structure creates a sense of security, and this includes physical security. For example, Theraplay places a high emphasis on making sure that the child cannot get hurt through the activities and also talks about this and demonstrates it to the child. For example, when preparing the child to karate-chop a sheet of newspaper, the therapist first checks how long the child's arm is and demonstrates that there is no risk of hitting the adult who is holding the newspaper. Marking the boundaries of the child's body is an important structuring element, and this is done in concrete terms, counting the child's toes, checking the length of the child's arms, fingers, legs, and smile and comparing them, drawing an outline of the child's body on a large sheet of paper—all these activities help develop the child's sense of self.

As Jukka Mäkelä said at the conference, the goal is to create a setting that engenders a sense of security, for example by being a "soft nest". Theraplay relies on familiar items that are found in most homes: cotton balls, soap bubbles, hand lotion, newspapers, feathers, balloons, etc. This element of familiarity should be established from the outset. The structure is established by means of rapid shifts, activities, and transitions. In any kind of therapy, it is essential to make sure that the experiences offer a sense of closure, and that the therapist conveys a single, coherent message from start to finish. This gives the child the experience that "I have the capacity to be good at something; I have the capacity to do well." This, in a sense, establishes an alternative to the controlling attachment pattern that especially disorganised children, who have been exposed to neglect and abuse, tend to develop.

The disorganised attachment pattern is profoundly destructive for psychological development, and the therapist has to relieve the child of this need for control by showing the child a different world where it is safe and feels good to be controlled by another person during these shared moments. The structure offers experiences that the child would not dare to pursue alone: for example, psychophysical experiences of good emotions. The therapist has to guess what the child needs and is able to handle, and, in this sense, the therapist is always taking risks. Misattunements are unavoidable and necessary, because they are a way of contributing something new by offering the corrective experience of having misattunements repaired. The way in which the child sits or is supported to sit, and the way in which the child's movements are created or expanded, give rise to emotions. In a sense, posture and movement precede emotions, and these factors can, therefore, be used to promote the emergence of new emotions. Change can also stem from making the child wait before acting: for example, if the therapist says, "Let's see if you can pop that soap bubble—1 . . . 2 . . . 3!" This intensifies the emotion. Waiting means being strong and competent, just as stopping instantly while play-fencing or engaging in other high-intensity activities also creates an emotional experience of personal strength.

Structure is important because a well-ordered world makes it safe to be curious, and curiosity is a basic feature of being a child. As adults, we cannot promise the child safety and security in this world, but we can create a safe microcosm. Creating a moment, a tiny world that is safe, enhances the child's capacity for trust.

In one of the video clips in Haldor Øvreeide's presentation, we saw a new foster mother who was trying to build an attachment with the infant that she was going to care for. In commenting on the video, Haldor Øvreeide used the term "intrusion" a few times to describe the foster mother's attempts to make contact. Later, Jukka Mäkelä reflected on the relevance of creating a structure that enables the child both to follow initiatives and to take the lead, and he argued that this kind of "intrusion" is quite essential. Haldor Øvreeide replied that he agreed that intrusion is necessary, but that the adult has to be careful not to go *too* far. Jukka Mäkelä commented that sometimes the good parent or therapist does things that are slightly "too much", but that is not necessarily problematic: Parents, therapists, and other adults are also entitled to initiative, just as the child is. What we saw in the video was that the child initially expresses, "I'm not so sure about this," through her body language, but this only lasted a few seconds, then she was able to process the experience and now seemed to say, again through body language and mimicry, "In fact, now that I've processed it, actually I *am* interested." Haldor Øvreeide mentioned that the beautiful thing about the clip was to see how the carer, with whom the child was already familiar, was able to support the child in exploring the foster mother, who was new to the child. Thus, the familiar person served as a secure base for the child and helped the child explore this novel experience. We return to this clip and some reflections on it in Chapter Eight.

Jukka Mäkelä pointed out that one of the important, non-specific factors is to make sure that there is something—the relationship, the structure, or the setting—that supports the child well enough to feel secure in following another person's initiatives and to contribute his or her own initiatives. In other words, it is essential to provide a secure structure or setting that frames the child's experiences and engagements and to notice and follow the child's initiative in order to discover what it means and add one's own.

## The importance of nurturing

As mentioned in Mäkelä and Hart's chapter on Theraplay (Hart, 2011), calming and nurturing activities make the world seem safe, predictable, warm, and secure and shows the child that the adult is a source of safety and stability. All children need nurturing to feel valuable and cared for, and all children need to have their stress levels reduced, to be soothed, to feel loved. When children receive care, they form a positive internal working model that lets them know that "I am worth loving, the world is a good place to be, other people are looking after me, and I am not alone." When the child grows older, there is a greater emphasis on the shared experience of sitting together, for example, sharing a pleasant experience, but still the core is that of sharing. The purpose of nurturing in therapy is to meet previously unmet needs from earlier stages of development.

A secure and empathic relationship establishes an emotional context where the child feels secure enough to be able to handle optimal stress levels. The feeling of attachment reduces anxiety and offers emotional protection in stressful situations. The therapist mimics the positive mirroring that parents offer their children under normal circumstances.

The parent–infant relationship contains many nurturing activities: The child is nursed, cradled, embraced, and comforted, to mention a few examples. These activities are soothing and play a crucial role in building a secure relationship. The parent foresees the child's needs and conveys the message that she understands and thinks about the child. By experiencing that there is a caring adult nearby when needed, the child gradually develops the capacity to internalise the carer's soothing function and learns how to carry out these functions along when the carer is not present.

Nurturing includes all the things that mothers do to alleviate the child's fear of being abandoned in a hostile world: a soft tone of voice, gentle but firm touch, care for injuries and scratches, and a loving facial expression. These elements let the helpless child know that he or she is going to be carried into life, guided and protected on his or her path through the many dangers that all living beings are hard-wired to expect.

Touch is an important theme in Theraplay, and at the conference this was the source of much debate; the topic is addressed later in this chapter. Jukka Mäkelä emphasised that when touch has been an element in connection with abuse, as is often the case with children who have an attachment disorder, touch has to be addressed with a high degree of sensitivity and self-awareness and with a focus on both transference and countertransference issues. To avoid using touch means abandoning the child to him/herself in a tough world, where the only reliable source of pleasure and joy is to be found individu-ally, in isolation—which is likely to feed addiction issues.

Jukka Mäkelä pointed out that there are two basic types of touch, both of which can be both nurturing and challenging. The light, feathery touch, which is almost like a tickle, is activating and stimu-lating. For example, parents often tickle their child in order to make the child laugh. In Theraplay, this kind of touch is used very rarely and only in clear agreement with the child: "Is it nice, do you like it?" The other kind of touch is a steady, rhythmic, deep touch that calms the child down by sending signals to deep-seated centres in the brain that increase oxytocin levels and, thus, the feeling of well-being in another person's company. This kind of touch is often used and is also taught to the parents as part of Theraplay. Most children who go into therapy need a high degree of external support to regulate their internal state, and deep touch is a good way of reducing stress and increasing their capacity for social engagement.

At the conference, Jukka Mäkelä explained that the purpose of touch in Theraplay is to recreate the psychophysical experience of receiving pleasure that humans share with all other animals. As humans, we are animals who need to find pleasure in interactions, pleasure in engaging, and pleasure in digesting. A wide variety of emotional mechanisms, which activate neurochemicals such as oxy-tocin and endorphins, give us the capacity for social engagement and the positive reward it offers. If this capacity is untapped and is, instead, transferred to solitary activities, as mentioned above, it can lead to problems with addiction. In a sense, the circuits that are supposed to be used for social engagement are hijacked by an addictive cycle. Jukka Mäkelä is convinced that giving pleasure in interactions offers some degree of protection against addiction and substance abuse. The therapist needs to be aware that it is difficult for children who have suffered severe neglect to maintain contact when they are relaxing. During the therapy session, it might be necessary to acknowledge the trust that the child shows: for example, by telling the child how impressed one is at how good the child is at accepting nurturing, relaxing, or closing his or her eyes and simply having something sweet in his/her mouth; telling the child how nice it is to see his or her ability to enjoy the interaction. It is important for the child to develop a sense that the therapist and, not least, the parents, appreciate and have feelings for the child, that they are pleased with the child's successes, and that they will provide support when the child encounters obstacles.

Jukka Mäkelä described how the child should be surrounded by a sense of security that is based on sensitivity. This involves an expanded use of touch where the therapist uses touch to maintain physical contact with the child and read the child's signals. The therapist also draws on scientific knowledge about calming touch, which means making sure that the touch is deep enough, and that it is slow, rhythmic, and pleasant and gives the child the experience of meaning and contact with others that activates the insula, a deep-seated brain structure that is involved, among other functions, in registering pain stimuli and integrating sensory modalities such as taste and smell.

A key topic in the panel debate was the use of touch in Jukka Mäkelä's therapy clips: for example, with Matias, the eight-year-old boy with an attachment disorder. The video shows him sitting with the boy on his lap, with some pillows between himself and the child, and massaging his arms and feet with oil. Eia Asen said that much of what Jukka Mäkelä does with the children in therapy would not be possible in the UK; specifically, therapists are not allowed to touch children. He said that it would be a serious issue, for example, to massage a child, even if the parents were present, since it could lead to allegations of sexual abuse. However, that does not stop the staff at the Marlborough Family Service from getting close to children. He said that he liked Jukka Mäkelä's idea of encircling the child; here he referred to a clip from Jukka Mäkelä's video presentation, where a female therapist comes close to a child with autism so suddenly that the child is startled and surprised, which produces a present moment.

Eia Asen considers this element of surprise, or of unpredictability, an important non-specific factor, as it offers an element that raises the level of activation and allows something new to happen.

Questions from the audience concerned how to make sure that the child is not overwhelmed by the therapist's presence and touch. Jukka Mäkelä's answer was "By being there. By knowing that I am a tremendous challenge to him and continuously asking, 'Is this OK? Are you tolerating this?'" Referring to the clip where he lifts the eight-year-old Matias on to a bed, Jukka Mäkelä explained that as he does this he checks whether Matias is permitting it. Because of the physical contact, Jukka Mäkelä can tell that Matias is not freezing, and neither is he going limp in the sense of acting like a passive victim. Matias assists, and this offered an initial indication of what was possible in the contact, and what was not. The physical contact provides an additional source of information, because the body is constantly communicating. On one level, of course, Matias was overwhelmed, but, on another level, he raised his hand right away when Jukka Mäkelä offered him his hand. As Peter Levine commented, Matias's adaptive capacity was challenged, and the only way to challenge someone's adaptive capacity is to challenge the zone of proximal development. Much of Jukka Mäkelä's work is about how to build an engagement that might seem like a confrontation, but which gives the child space to develop.

Jukka Mäkelä was present in the moment and ready to accept a "No". The therapist has to be able to sense that he or she is on the verge of something that is traumatic and avoid overstepping that particular boundary. This involves being able to read the child's signals and offer good experiences where the child can feel safe and act with curiosity. This lets the therapist pull the child into the comfort zone, even if it is an unfamiliar one.

Peter Levine added that the climate in the USA is characterised by a similar hysteria about touching, as in the UK. For that reason, he has stopped showing videos that include very intimate touch. In his assessment, this state of affairs speaks to the pathology of the society. Peter Levine described how, even when he is watching children play or if he takes a picture of his godchild, who is three and a half years old, playing with her friends, his friends will say, "Don't do that. You could get arrested!" He saw this as a sad development and was pleased to see that Theraplay has the courage and the freedom to explore the potential of appropriate touch. Jukka Mäkelä responded that Theraplay is used widely in some parts of the USA, and there has never been an allegation of sexual impropriety against any of the hundreds of therapists who use Theraplay. He added that in the UK, the adoption centre Family Futures also uses touch as part of Theraplay. However, Jukka Mäkelä has encountered the issue in Finland, too, where touching is considered completely off limits in psychoanalysis, for example, and he has often been asked if it is really appropriate. The concern about how the child and the parents construe the use of touch is very relevant, but, in Jukka Mäkelä's assessment, without these corrective experiences of touch, the child might continue to construe adults and closeness to adults as something associated with abuse. The child needs to learn the difference between appropriate and inappropriate ways of being with others, and one of the goals of Theraplay is to show children an appropriate way of touching.

Haldor Øvreeide pointed out that in relation to sexual abuse there are several problems at play. As an example, he mentioned "grooming", where a paedophile, over time, establishes a relationship of trust with a child, perhaps including the people around the child, where the child gradually learns to accept the abuse as "normal". As this abusive process is based on intimacy, he expressed some concern that the pleasant touch that is seen in Theraplay could activate grooming processes. He described having seen videos made by paedophiles who had groomed a child and seen the child freeze when the actual act of abuse begins.

Eia Asen agreed with Jukka Mäkelä that the child needs corrective experiences. He argued that it was necessary to have the non-abusive parent or other trusted adults from the wider family network to offer these experiences. The Marlborough Family Service does not use parallel sessions, where the parents watch the therapist with the child, so, instead, they try to enable the parents to provide these corrective experiences. Peter Levine mentioned that because touch gives such an important proprioceptive experience through the insula structure of the brain, he sometimes uses beanbags where the child has one beanbag behind them and one on top of them; when he pushes a little bit the child will feel the weight of that and push back in response.

When asked whether it was more acceptable for a female than a male psychotherapist to touch the child, Peter Levine said that it probably would be more acceptable, while Eia Asen did not think that made any difference, as the UK had seen horrendous scandals with female nursery staff who had committed sexual abuse. In conclusion to this dialogue, we pointed out the paradox at play here. The importance of physical contact is clearly documented, for example in Uvnäs-Moberg's (1997a,b, 1998) work on oxytocin (a hormone that supports the sense of security, and which is produced in response to calm, firm touch and gentle contact) and moulding (the child's ability to "melt" into the carer's embrace). On the one hand, therapists need to find a way to stimulate the proprioceptive sense to activate the oxytocin response, and, on the other hand, they have to proceed with caution, because we live in a complex world. Solving this conundrum requires creative approaches.

## Following and matching the child's responses

Right from the outset of a therapy session, the therapist has to take charge and act as the proverbial caravan leader. At the conference, Jukka Mäkelä explained that Theraplay has a very deliberate approach to issues of closeness and distance in therapy. Wherever the child's zone of proximal development lies, the therapist has to create an interaction where the child feels seen, acknowledged and met in a mutual or symmetrical relationship. In therapy sessions, Theraplay therapists focus their attention on the child and/or the parents, and they get in very close. As psychotherapists, they know that this is confrontational, and that it is, therefore, important to modulate the impact. The goal is to try to make very rapid changes, for example, by making it clear that "now we are presenting you with a challenge". The therapist tries to let the child know that the therapy experience offers a different world than the one the child is familiar with—a world where it is possible to be close to another person, face to face, and still feel safe. It is a challenge for the therapist to establish a sense of security, since, of course, one cannot simply tell the child to feel safe. Jukka Mäkelä said that he was surprised when he first began to learn about Theraplay, because he had been trained in classic child psychotherapy, where the trust is established very gradually. Seeing

Peter Levine's work, much of what he saw was immediately recognisable, especially the incident in Levine's video where the mother is holding the baby, while Levine is positioned quite close to them, and the baby begins to play with Peter Levine's finger. Jukka Mäkelä explained that he had done exactly the same thing countless times, where the child responds to the fingers. He had enjoyed seeing Peter Levine's way of building on that, for example by taking the intensity up and down with the rattle. The point where the baby pushes with his legs is so important, and it is worthwhile for the child to do it over and over again.

Jukka Mäkelä wondered whether it is actually the child or the therapist who is carrying out the therapy when they have established a strong alliance. He referred specifically to Peter Levine's video where he supports Johnny's traumatic experience of the drowning accident, and both Johnny and Susie take active part in the intervention. Jukka Mäkelä mentioned how nice it was to see how many shared consciousnesses were involved, how Susie took part in the therapy, and how Johnny worked through his part, and then how Peter Levine was able to discuss the incident with both of them at once, except when Susie needed more focused attention, and Johnny left the room. In presenting the video, Peter Levine had explained that Johnny left the room because he probably needed some space, but in fact Jukka Mäkelä thought the boy might have left because he wanted to make room for Susie to work through her trauma. Peter Levine said that this was a fascinating possibility, adding that he was always struck by the magic of what happens and the things that really cannot be explained. Haldor Øvreeide commented that the reason why it is meaningful to ask who is actually doing the therapy, the child or the therapist, is that the therapist has managed to connect with the child or the children on relevant issues. Once this connection has been made, the children make the process their own. Peter Levine added that it is often in that first part of a minute where this is either achieved or not; however, if the connection is not made, the key is simply to recalibrate and try again. It is all about the therapist's capacity to capture the present moment and allow it to unfold.

Haldor Øvreeide pointed to the important role of the co-operative process between the child and the parent or therapist; this is a crucial condition for the adult's ability to follow and match the child's responses. There are certain basic interactive capacities with which the child meets the world, and which therapists and parents need to understand and bring into their relationships with the child. Previously, Haldor Øvreeide has used the term "transactional", but today he prefers the concept of "co-operation", because the process is really about developmental collaboration. It is not simply a transactional process of give and take. This is a creative process where the therapist puts in something new without knowing exactly what the outcome is going to be. It is crucial to take a co-operative approach to this process. Haldor Øvreeide underlined the importance of acting in accordance with the child's basic capacities in order to attune with the child's specific experiences and offer developmental support. The therapist can build on these capacities and adjust them in various ways. If necessary, the therapist can support an adaptive deconstruction of certain ways of relating to the world and, in turn, support the reconstruction of individual and interpersonal patterns, not least the life narratives that that hamper or disrupt development. Haldor Øvreeide summarised three general focal points in this process: being in the dialogue or the process, understanding or having a perspective on the power situation that the child lives in, that is, the regulation of roles and power management, and having ideas about the intended outcome of the therapeutic effort. With regard to the outcome, Haldor Øvreeide described two levels: one level is about creating more constructive patterns of interaction between parent and child; the other level has to do with meaning-making narratives that promote the development of the parents' self-respect and their respect for the child.

## Summary

In this chapter, we have addressed the relationship between therapist and child and discussed the importance of embracing one's authority and the asymmetrical responsibility while also doing everything possible to maintain a symmetrical relationship with the child. Peter Levine, Jukka Mäkelä, Haldor Øvreeide, and Eia Asen all emphasised the importance of really seeing the child and of embracing the asymmetrical responsibility while maintaining a symmetrical relationship. Inspired by Eia Asen's work, Jukka Mäkelä pointed out that many parents fail to understand how their image and perception of the child affect their relationship with the child as well as the child's actions and behaviour. A therapist has to be willing to take risks, which requires a keen awareness and profound understanding of one's own effect on others. The therapist should also demonstrate to both the child and the parents how one person can have a profound impact on another person. This involves modelling behaviour and functioning as a role model, not only to the parents but also to the child, in a way that demonstrates that we all have an impact on each other. This also means that therapists should not simply try to copy other therapists' interventions. Every therapist should develop his or her own authentic style and pay attention to the way in which his or her interventions affect the child and/or parents.

# CHAPTER EIGHT

# Enacting the child's feelings in the psychotherapeutic process

"When we give the child self-organising agency we have to expect the situation to be outside the adult's control. We have to expect a different outcome than we had originally intended, because we have given agency to the other, in this case the child"

(Haldor Øvreeide)

I n a chapter on regulation in the relationship between infant and carer, Sander (1977) describes his systemic perspective and points out how there is always a natural polarity between rhythms that ensure adaptation and attachment and states that disrupt rhythms and produce uncertainty, variation, and differences, and which require reorganisation after a painful disruption and disorganisation. Instead of avoidance, protection, and withdrawal, it is the ability to meet uncertainty and disruption that ensures the continuation of the creative process in the development of the nervous system. Thus, as humans, we strive with all our might for safety and security, yet it is our ability to tolerate and endure uncertainty and disruption that enables us to continue our development. This confronts us with an apparent paradox: out of random occurrences must come order; out of uncertainty must come knowledge; out of chaos must come a creative capacity. Sander concludes that being close to development means being close to the stress, anxiety, loss, and loneliness that are caused by the painful childhood moments characterised by recurrent disruption. This, according to Sander, frames the creative process in life.

Recent studies of the human cortisol metabolism and attachment behaviour have confirmed that a well-regulated emotional relationship characterised by open and receptive communication provides a regulation system of more inclusive adaptation that is associated with reduced cortisol levels in response to mild stress factors.

Moments of meeting alter the implicit relational expectations in both parties and signal an opening for expanding new initiatives. Moments of meeting create the potential for expanding new types of shared experiences and a new level of mutual and receptive regulation. Intersubjective moments of meeting are experienced and represented in implicit relational knowledge and might or might not become the object of interpretation. In any circumstance, these moments of meeting enable more complex ways of being with others.

As mentioned earlier, emotional balance and attunement do not follow the same course of development as our cognitive skills. Emotional skills stem from living life here and now within the context of human interactions that we learn on an unconscious level. We share experiences as they occur, and our way of being with each other unfolds in the moment, before the experience has been transferred or rephrased in words. The desire to feel attachment with others is important for the formation of relations and also plays a key role in the psychotherapy process (Hart, 2012). In this chapter, we take a closer look at what constitutes the non-specific experiences that vitalise and enable these moments of meeting.

### *Synchronisered attachment experiences are created through affective attunement*

In the chapter "Affect attunement", Stern (1984) describes that a characteristic of attunement is that there is a match that is not an imitation.

This match is largely cross-modal, which means that the channel or modality of expression used by the mother to match the infant is different from the channel or modality used by the infant. According to Stern, what is being matched is not the other person's behaviour *per se*, but, rather, some aspect of an internal feeling state. The reference for the match appears to be the internal state, not the external behavioural event. This means that affect attunement is a particular form of intersubjectivity that concerns interaffectivity.

Stern uses the term affect attunement to mean a behaviour that expresses the emotional character of a shared state without actually imitating the exact behaviour. Affect attunement is needed to shift the focus of attention to the inside, to the quality of feeling that is being shared, and it is used to commune or indicate sharing of internal states. Attunement renders feelings. The largest single reason for performing an attunement is "to be with" the infant in what Stern calls "interpersonal communion", which means to participate together, or to share in another's experience. The other's internal state is experienced through attributes or qualities of perception, that is, through vitality, degree of pleasure, level of activation, and the discrete category of the other's affective sensation. For example, when we see another person's arm gesture, we may grasp the perceptual properties of rapid acceleration, speed, fullness of display, and rapid deceleration, that is, a quality of feeling or a form of vitality. Attunements are experienced as an uninterrupted process and appear with feeling qualities such as explosions, fadings, rushings, etc. Attunements are dynamic, kinetic feeling qualities that correspond to the constantly variable ubiquitous organic processes of being alive. Attunement behaviour begins as soon as social interactions occur. Around the age of nine months, infants begin to cross an interpersonal threshold that makes attunement a completely different experience. At this time, infants come to the gradual but momentous discovery that they have a mind, and that other people have separate minds, and that the child is able to sense both at the same time. The child learns that what can be attuned to with the carer is sharable and becomes the stuff of intimacy. The infant's sense of self as "reflected" by the parents will be shaped by the history of past and present attunements and misattunements, making the attunement process a helpful therapeutic tool. In other words, attunement processes drive the intersubjective development processes.

## Implicit relational knowledge

Lyons-Ruth (1998) has described how interactional processes from birth onward give rise to a form of procedural knowledge regarding how to do things with intimate others. In the therapy process, the child's and the therapist's unconscious, or implicit, relational knowledge intersect to create an intersubjective field that includes reasonably accurate ideas about the other's way of being with others. As mentioned earlier, this intersubjective field consists of many present moments and gives rise to new dyadic interaction in the form of new adaptive acts and shared intersubjective recognition. These moments of meeting enable new forms of agency and shared experiences that can be expressed and expanded. They make it possible to direct one's attention at oneself and one's inner sensations, thus expanding self-awareness. It is through the eyes of others that we learn to see ourselves.

Some of our shared behaviour with others is encoded as rule-based procedural representations, generally described in individual skills such as knowing how to ride a bicycle, but which are also at the heart of how to do things with others. The Boston Change Study Group termed this unconscious, implicit, or procedural knowledge about how to do things with others: "implicit relational knowledge". This develops long before language, and it continues to guides our personal interactions throughout life, but it is not language-based and is not automatically translated into verbal form. Thus, some areas of the child's implicit relational knowledge may be subject to verbal articulation and interpretation, but it mainly operates outside our verbal awareness.

An authentic, or "genuine", relationship that emerges in the intersubjective field unfolds in the intersection between both parties' implicit relational knowledge and includes authentic personal engagement and an accurate sense of the individual's current "ways of being with" others. A "moment of meeting" is an event that reshapes the child's implicit relational knowledge as a result of an altered intersubjective field between the child and therapist. It is co-constructed and requires a unique contribution from both parties with a specific recognition of the other's subjective reality.

At the conference, Jukka Mäkelä mentioned how, in traditional psychiatry and psychology circles, he frequently found that he had to defend his claim that experiences in themselves are sufficient for maturing certain parts of the central nervous system. To develop self-regulation competences in relation to emotional experiences and to develop strengths and experiences of mastery, we need concrete experiences with another person. The present moments arise through shared experiences and cannot be achieved by the rational brain. The regulation of increasing and decreasing states of tension, activation and calming, lets us expand our emotional experiences. The most activating feeling for any animal is surprise. When something new and different happens, we shut everything else out for a moment and enter into an intense state where we invest a huge amount of emotion in a single experience. As the next step, we use repetition to make experiences feel safe. We repeat an activity over and over again to make sure that the child can safely engage in the experiences and move on, ideally before the child begins to feel bored. This is one of the ways through which the child learns arousal regulation.

### Attunement processes and arousal regulation

At the conference, Peter Levine commented that, in his experience, ADHD is not due to hyper-arousal but, instead, due to a child's attempts at keeping the energy going to avoid experiencing a psychological shut-down, which is a terrifying feeling of being trapped. When he works with children who have ADHD symptoms, he never tries to make them relax, because that risks pushing them into immobility. First, they have to build the necessary resources, which was demonstrated in the Theraplay clip with Matias when he pushed Jukka Mäkelä, who flew backwards, kicking his feet in the air. Children love that, they laugh, even though they know it is an act, it is make-believe. Peter Levine suggested a different approach, saying to the child, "Now can you push the smallest amount and really feel inside of you where that comes from?" This will help the child move out of immobility without quickly going back into it. To illustrate, Jukka Mäkelä demonstrated an exercise with Peter Levine, where he asked Peter Levine to stand face to face with him as they built a "hand tower", one hand on top of the next, etc. Jukka Mäkelä regulated the pace with his voice, using volume, tone, and tempo, spelling out the turns, saying "Peter, Jukka, Peter, Jukka, Peter, Jukka, Peter, Jukka.

That's really good. Let's start going down . . ." Gradually, Jukka Mäkelä's voice became softer, and the pace slowed down. Then Jukka Mäkelä said very softly, Now, Peter, I want you to do it with just one finger, like that: your finger, my finger (*whispering*) and now, close your eyes . . . Right. OK. You feel that?"

Peter Levine commented that this was a perfect example of what he was talking about. To further illustrate his point about experiences from within, he asked to demonstrate an exercise with Jukka Mäkelä. He used the trust pendulum, where the person is asked to dare to lean into someone else's arms, and which challenges the child's capacity for following. Peter Levine demonstrated with Jukka how tiny variations in touch produce a different experience and an internal sense of motion. This produces a very different effect and proprioceptive stimulation, and has a more profound effect on the cerebellar circuits.

At the conference, a member of the audience asked how immobil-isation and dissociation is expressed in infants and how to tell when the infant is unable to engage in attunement processes. Referring to the psychologist René Spitz's film (1952) from an orphanage, Peter Levine described how some of the orphans in the film are clearly not psychologically present; they have a blank expression and do not relate to their environment, but simply stare into emptiness. He described the immediate feeling that this produces as absolutely heart-breaking. It is an abnormal expression of absence and vacancy, since children are normally constantly exploring and learning. Jukka Mäkelä mentioned an example of a three-year-old girl who sometimes displayed a puzzling physical change that was felt as a temperature difference in her hands that the adult could feel when holding her hands. There was also a change in her face, perhaps a pallor, but what was most noticeable was that the small muscles in her face stopped moving. In a way, she was with them, interacting, but she was not present. Then they changed what they did by noticing when this occurred, stopping and saying, "Oh, there's something going on now," and then working on those moments. The dissociation is evident in a sense that the child seems absent. Although the child might be looking at one's face, the gaze is vacant and empty.

This sparked another question from the audience about the shut-down response. The question specifically referred to the example of a nine-year-old child whose parents are divorcing. The boy participates in a group, and although he is present in the group, he is emotionally

"flat", with a face that lacks tone and expression. Peter Levine responded that the shut-down system is a typical defence response, and
that it is necessary to proceed more carefully with that sort of defence
than with the more active defence system, because it is so easy to go
past the child's threshold and cause further shut-down. The therapists
will need to observe very carefully to see if it is possible to find active
responses, such as the play-fencing that Jukka Mäkelä demonstrated
in Theraplay sessions. That will activate the body and help the boy
receive proprioceptive feedback to help him escape the shut-down.

Eia Asen added that, in his experience, children are not always in
a dissociative state, so the therapist's job is to create a connection,
perhaps through a third object or a game, that brings the child back to
life. It is the therapist's responsibility to find what it will take to make
that connection, and Peter Levine mentioned that it is important to
work with the child's arousal level as a key present moment to help
bring the child out of the dissociative state. As we added at the conference, when the face is perceived as expressionless, there *is*, in fact, a
facial expression, but this expression is not connected to the micro-
rhythms of the interaction. As Eia Asen pointed out, dissociation is not
either present or absent, it can be present in varying degrees; sometimes the dissociative state is quite severe, sometimes it is less severe,
and it is the therapist's job to seize the moments when the child is
more open to interaction and build on that opportunity. In other
words, the key is to identify the resources or the development process
in the zone of proximal development and build on that.


## Accepting feelings by following the developmental process

To illustrate the notion of following the development process, Haldor
Øvreeide showed a video clip from the Danish observation and treatment centre Skodsborg Observations- og Behandlingshjem, which
we mentioned briefly in Chapter Seven. The clip gives an impression
of the balancing act that carers undertake in relation to children's
development.

The film showed a woman who was going to be the foster mother
of an infant girl. She was meeting the child for the first time, together
with a carer from the childcare facility where the child had been
placed. The film showed the first dramatic moments of this meeting.

The child was very familiar with the carer, who brought in the child, looked at the child, and then smiled at the future foster mother. The child looked at the new face, then turned away, hiding her own face, while the foster mother put the experience into words: "Did you get shy?" thus accepting and supporting the child's withdrawal. The child looked up again, monitoring the foster mother's actions, and while she was still clinging to her familiar carer, she held out her hand. The carer took the child's hand, and both the carer and the foster mother now looked at the child. Suddenly, the child withdrew, then turned back to face the foster mother before she again buried her face in the carer's shoulder and chest. The foster mother reached out, and the child took her hand, while the carer watched. Then, suddenly, it was enough! The child turned away, and the carer supported and balanced her withdrawal, and, thus, the foster mother's approach was rejected. Her initiative was too much, and the child withdrew. Instead of respecting the withdrawal, the foster mother continued her contact initiative, while the carer, who knew the child, accepted the child's withdrawal. She held the child close, saying "That's fine, that's fine," thus also helping the foster mother manage her emotions. The child sensed that the foster mother came in too close, but the carer helped her. The child reached out, the foster mother leaned in, and the child again took the initiative to reach out. The child wanted to explore by repeating what had happened before, and the carer watched what was going on. The foster mother reached out, enclosing the child's hand fully in both her hands, but, oh, again it was too much! The child pulled back her hand. The foster mother now held out one hand, but again, the child withdrew. The foster mother invited again, but the child was reluctant. The carer read the child and saw that this encounter was too much for her, and said, "Just say hello." The foster mother said, "Where's your nose," reaching out and touching the child's nose, while the carer watched the child's reaction closely. The foster mother said, "Where's my nose?" The child reached out and touched the foster mother's nose, and they had eye contact. The foster mother smiled, the carer looked at her and shared the smile.

Haldor Øvreeide explained that the staff at Skodsborg was committed to helping the future foster mother co-regulate with the child. They spent two months at the centre to help the child achieve good co-regulation with the foster mother, and eventually the child accepted her as the main carer. The film illustrated how important it is for the child to receive this support in connection with such a dramatic change. Haldor Øvreeide explained that he had chosen the clip because it offers an excellent illustration of the general process that carers or therapists engage in with infants.

Haldor Øvreeide characterises the developmentally supportive dialogue as a special combination of dialogue processes, social roles, meaning making, and narratives where the adult makes sense of the world together with the child. The carer has to be able to read the child as accurately as possible when the child unfolds his or her capacities in physical and mental states, while also being able to monitor him/herself and mark the possible growth moments that the child might need at different age levels. This is a complicated process and a cultural project that includes the child's individual developmental processes. In the developmental dialogue, the parent must be motivated by an intention: "I want something for my child." The carer enters into the developmental project with certain ideas, which may have a cultural focus or a more individual intention of helping the child in some way. However, the developmental dialogue is also motivated by the process—it is a human interaction that motivates itself as it falls into a specific, well-functioning process, where the adult is motivated to be present. Haldor Øvreeide mentioned that he sees this motivation at play when the children he works with wish to stay in the therapy room, because the process is providing something that is motivating in itself. He often finds that parents are in a state of "I have to . . ."; they are not motivated by the process itself, but by this sense that they have to do something, which seems tiresome and fatiguing. This underlines the importance of creating an engaging process with the child in the therapy room.

To demonstrate his point, Haldor Øvreeide showed a video sequence of Ane Kristine, who was about five weeks old in the first clip. She was with her mother, who was changing her nappy, washing her, and dressing her. They had good eye contact, and the mother was offering the child her face and her voice, speaking baby talk, touching and stroking the little girl's stomach, saying all these important things and giving the girl space to organise and to find the mother. The mother touched the little girl's legs, the girl's eyes wandered, then she refocused on the mother, they had eye contact, touch, support, and she turned her face towards the mother again. The mother responded with, "Oh, you're beautiful; everything's fine; you're wonderful, yes you are." Ane Kristine focused on her mother, registering her mother and then lifted her chin twice, and the mother responded, "Yes, hello—you want to tell me something?" The mother interpreted the two chin movements as "Ah, you want to say something," attributing mental motivation to Ane Kristine. Another sound from the baby: "Errch." The mother was right, there was an impulse; when Ane Kristine focused on her mother's face and engaged in the relationship she seemed to have an internal motivation of bringing something to the relationship—she wanted to say something. Often, this kind of sequence would be labelled as mirroring, but Haldor Øvreeide thought that this term was misleading. The child has an intrinsic capacity to say something, which constitutes a self-organised and self-produced invitation to communication. Thus, what is played out in this type of incident is the principle of self-organisation, or agency, which is quite different from mirroring.

The film clip continued: the mother asked Ane Kristine, "Would you like some cod liver oil?" The girl responded with a happy facial expression. The mother moved out of the relationship and instead checked how the girl's navel was healing. This meant that Ane Kristine was left to herself, and she responded by making an insistent, frustrated sound to indicate that she wanted to keep the relationship with the mother going; this demonstrates that the girl had the capacity to express and repair a misattunement. When stress occurs in the communication process, the first thing the child does is to try to show him/herself with even greater intensity or impact. So, here we saw a disruption and a repair, as the mother returned her attention to the child, saying, "Yes, there you are!" The mother now wanted to give Ane Kristine some cod liver oil and reached for the bottle. The girl's gaze followed the mother's hand—what Daniel Stern calls "moving along" towards the moment of meeting. The mother attempted to regulate her actions to enable a moment of meeting, and the mother and Ane Kristine had already established a pattern based on expectations that had sprung from the previous incidents. Within this pattern, they both did their best to create new interactive moments. Ane Kristine expected a nice mother and nice experiences and expected the mother to respect her self-organisation. The mother usually makes pleasant sounds, her hands are soft . . . that was what Ane Kristine was expecting, but what did she get? A teaspoon of cod liver oil! We saw that Ane Kristine had an expectation based on previous

experiences, but the moment that occurred had a very different quality: "My self-regulation was completely blocked, and I had to accept
what my mother just did to me!" The mother said, "Yes, you're a good
girl, it's over now." Ane Kristine withdrew, her eyes wandered, the
mother tried to re-establish contact, but Ane Kristine looked away and
withdrew. "You were such a good girl, and now it's over," said the
mother, but Ane Kristine withdrew from the interaction and was no
longer looking at the mother. The mother again tried to re-establish
contact but failed. The mother respected the withdrawal and stayed
with Ane Kristine until the girl had recuperated, and they resumed
their interaction a few moments later.

In another clip, we saw Ane Kristine looking at a play of light on
the bathroom wall while the mother was changing her nappy. From
her body movements, she appeared to be reaching for the specks of
light on the wall, squirming eagerly. Haldor pointed out that Ane
Kristine showed the same impulse as in the previous clip with the
mother's face; she wanted to say something, contribute to the interaction. She turned her attention to the play of light and engaged in a sort
of interaction; she wanted to interact with the light, so she began to
move her whole body, but, of course, she could not reach the sun.
Then the mother came in and noticed that her daughter was looking
at the play of light on the wall. She said, "What are you looking at,"
while tapping her fingertips on the wall where the light was dancing.
In this way, she participated in Ane Kristine's lived moment and even
added something by drumming her fingers and making a sound with
her voice: "boop, boop, boop." Ane Kristine's attention to the moment
was intensified further, and we saw the mother looking at her intently
as if she were asking herself, "How is my child experiencing this
moment?" Perhaps this was one of the first examples of them sharing
the external world, but they did not share it in a passive way; it was
an active process where the mother shared the world with her child
and even added something new. For both of them, the process in
the present moment is, thus, about actively sharing the world and
adding something new. She added something that Ane Kristine found
relevant, and which maintained her attention. They were following
each other, and the mother added relevance. In the final clip with
Ane Kristine, the girl was very active and energetic. She had been
looking at something in the corner, and now the mother brought the
object into focus. She interpreted Ane Kristine's interest and looked

in the corner, saying, "Yes, you're a very clever girl," and Ane Kristine looked towards the corner again. She was squirming, shrieking, seeming excited and eager, and the mother read her intentions and brought the exciting part of the world to her: a bottle of soap. And not just the soap but also a bottle of moisturiser! Haldor Øvreeide was speculating that the girl might be thinking, "I have a very clever mother, she gives life to the world, and she always brings in new elements. It's nice, in colour, and she gives sound to the world," but also: "The world is full of disturbances, so now my father is coming in. There he is. OK. You disturbed a very nice moment, but anyway . . ."

The father came in, he was smiling, sat down, moved in close, said, "Heeey," with a soft, happy voice, and Ane Kristine gave him a smile. Haldor Øvreeide imagined that the girl was thinking, "I'll give you a smile and see what happens." The father said, "Are you going to have a bath?" He smiled. Ane Kristine returned her attention to the world and the moisturiser bottle. The father wanted to take part in the inter-action, and he wanted another smile. He reached for the moisturiser bottle, Ane Kristine opened her eyes, and he was holding the bottle in his hand, asking, "Is it a nice bottle?" This contribution was very different from the mother's. The mother was not asking but stating, "It's nice. It's a very nice bottle." But the father was passive here, and Ane Kristine looked as if she was saying, "Say something; tell me something; I don't understand you." But then she returned to the moisturiser and brought extra energy into the moment by opening her eyes wide, moving energetically, as if she was saying, "I want to play with it!" She turned to the father again, as if she was encouraging him to follow, but no, he did not follow! She went all out in a third attempt, raising her head up, lifting her hand, smiling, kicking, shrieking, and opening her eyes extra wide. But he failed to engage in the interaction, and then the girl looked at the camera operator, then back at her mother. At this point, she was three months old, and it was evident that she was attempting to organise the dialogue process around the item that she was interested in and in finding ways to develop in inter-actions with her parents. In this particular moment, the father was not as much help as he was in another, later moment. So, this is not about the person's sex; it is about knowing and reading the child in the moment. The mother and the child had been home all day, while the father had been away at work, so maybe for that reason he is more focused on the emotional aspect of the relationship, while Ane Kristine was more focused on exploring the world with her parents. Haldor Øvreeide commented that these video sequences showed the active unfolding child, and that understanding this developmental dialogue is absolutely crucial. The sequence illustrates the ideas that he bases his therapy on. The therapist is facing a creative, unfolding child and has to relate to the child in ways that are relevant to the child.

Eia Asen commented that he has observed Haldor Øvreeide's work several times, and that he admires the detailed attention he brings to even the most microscopic interactions, shifts, and changes. Much of this is based on following, which Haldor demonstrates both physically and verbally. He follows the child with his eyes, gets up and follows the child, returns with the child, etc. Eia Asen suggested that following, both physically and metaphorically, has to be one of the most important non-specific factors, along with relevance, which stimulates curiosity. He mentioned that Haldor Øvreeide does this, in part, by the questions he asks. For example, while Ane Kristine's mother brought in the new object, the father, by contrast, was more interested in stimulating Ane Kristine's curiosity in him than in following her. A good therapist has the ability to stimulate curiosity that matches what the child is interested in, and the best way of capturing a child's attention is following.

After Haldor Øvreeide's film clip, there was a question from the audience about whether the non-specific factors are the same as the factors that are considered *sine qua non* in psychotherapy, and whether they define action processes that are psychotherapeutic in nature. In response to this question, Haldor Øvreeide said that he had virtually lost track of the concept of psychotherapy. To him, the key focus has to be on developmental processes. Developmental arrest can occur for a number of reasons: for example, because one does not understand the child's individual factors, temperament, etc. There may also be developmental challenges that are present in the moment: for example, in connection with a divorce. In Haldor Øvreeide's opinion, the key is to offer developmental support, whether the situation is about therapy, or counselling, or some other context. The process has more to do with an understanding of children's development than with a particular method.

### Feed-forward systems

A "feed-forward" system prepares the parties for the next episode or action sequence. As an example of a feed-forward system, Haldor Øvreeide referred to the video of Ane Kristine. Already, at the age of five weeks, Ane Kristine had, in a sense, begun to establish a pattern for being with her mother, and she based her actions on expectations about what the next moment would bring. From the very first interaction, she had begun to construct a related expectation of the next moment. When this feed-forward process works well, it is easy for the parties to enter into the same pattern and to build on it. In the video, we saw how Ane Kristine looked at one thing, which the mother then brought into the interaction; this let them act together in relation to a shared object. They had a pattern, and it was obvious that they had done this before. Their interaction unfolded in a systematic, efficient, and developmental manner. In therapy, if the relationship is to develop into a co-operative pattern, the therapist should always be very aware of the first shared episodes, and how they are constructed. It is crucial to establish a positive feed-forward system. This involves establishing small attachment experiences, and, indeed, communication patterns can be viewed as an attachment system. The more relevant the therapist is to the child, the more the child will want to return to the therapist and use the therapeutic process to handle challenges or issues.

Haldor Øvreeide pointed out that Eia Asen's approach in the video with Akil was a brilliant example of breaking a feed-forward pattern that had been established between mother and child, based on trusting and knowing that they had the necessary resources to handle the change. He argued that therapists should dare to do this more often, but that, of course, they also have to be sure that they can support the family sufficiently and help them find new ways, as it takes time to establish a new relationship of trust. It was obviously crucial for Akil to be liberated and find the ability to move on, but, at the same time, he also needed his mother, and she needed time to adjust, as the blockage was very much hers and not Akil's.

### The five basic elements

Haldor Øvreeide described that in this process he relies on the five basic elements that were described on p. 110 in this volume: following, relevance, agency space, co-regulation, and hierarchy. When he sticks to these elements in his interactions with the child, the process keeps moving forward. The participants may take breaks, they might have to recreate the elements in the interaction, and it is not necessarily a smooth and flawless dance, but, by adhering to these basic approaches, therapists can make sure that they are able to keep the communication going. The adult senses the child's physical and mental states in somatic, perceptual, emotional, and cognitive terms. The carer has to be able to offer the child something that is relevant to him or her, or the child will withdraw, as we saw in the example with Ane Kristine and her father. Love is not enough; there has to be something of substance that will help the child develop. There also has to be room for the child's agency. This means that the adult has to provide time, physical and mental space, acknowledge the child's self-organising agency, and make room for, and accept, the child's responses. The adult must not only make room for the child's agency, but actively support it. The two parties engage in co-regulation, rhythm, and turn-taking. When we give the child self-organising agency we have to expect the situation to be outside the adult's control. We have to expect a different outcome than we had originally intended, because we have given agency to the other, in this case the child. Thus, the outcome will be outside our control. The final element is hierarchy; this implies that there is a responsible adult who takes a lead position and accepts the overall responsibility based on an intention of providing support.

## Summary

In this chapter, we have looked at developmental processes and the enlivening of the psychotherapy process. The therapeutic process and the most important condition for attunement is being with the child, which means having shared experiences. That is also what drives the therapy process. As Jukka Mäkelä pointed out, we have to share concrete experiences with someone else in order to develop our self-regulation capacity in relation to various emotional experiences and in order to develop our sense of strength and mastery. Present moments arise through shared experiences and through a regulation of rising and falling states of tension, which enable an expansion of emotional experiences. When something new and unusual happens, we shut everything else out for a moment and experience an intensity that is charged with a high degree of emotion. As Haldor Øvreeide pointed out, the child must be supported when dramatic changes occur, and it is crucial to create an engaging process with the child in the therapy room. The therapist is dealing with a creative child who expresses him/herself and needs to relate to the child in ways that are relevant to that child. Haldor Øvreeide refers to this as a developmentally supportive dialogue. Eia Asen added that this process requires following, both physically and verbally.

# CHAPTER NINE

# Magic and transformation

"All therapy is an archetype of the magical stranger—someone who comes in from the outside, works their magic, and then disappears from the person's life. It is interesting how much can be done in that relationship that doesn't really figure into any other relationships; it's not a transference relationship—it's a fairytale kind of thing"

(Peter Levine)

As described by Stern (2004), the therapy process involves acquiring new experiences, which do not repair the past, but are integrated into the nervous system. These changes in neural circuits make it possible to establish a new context where something new can emerge. The process has to be repeated over and over again to reinforce the neural circuits. In a sense, the past is transformed or restructured by being put together in a new way. New experiences are capable of rewriting the neural circuits that contained previous memory tracks. Thus, the therapy process, with its numerous present moments, leads to a rewriting of old history. The goal of the psychotherapy process is to find and restructure the child's strategies for regulating his or her mental and physical states. Affect regulation is part of the implicit memory system, and the regulation mechanisms are activated when a situation matches a prototype of a previous experience where this behaviour proved useful. For the psychotherapist, the goal is to activate the child's self-regulating capacity. In previous chapters, we have seen how self-regulating processes in the psychotherapy process develop through attunements and misattunements between therapist and child that unfold in present moments. Psychotherapy can offer a new model for the nature of close relationships and, ultimately, help child and parents reflect on events and their own emotions, behaviour patterns, etc.

In this chapter, we address the transformation process and the magical moments that generate transformation. We also discuss the need for the therapist to engage in risk-taking in this process.

## Therapy is child's play

As described in *Neuroaffektiv psykoterapi med børn* (Hart, 2011), engagement defines our central, personal, focused connection with another person. In the relationship between a parent and an infant, the parent has to notice what the infant is experiencing and help the child achieve an optimal arousal state. If the child is upset, the parent helps the child calm down; if the child is sleepy, the parent puts the child to bed; if the child is ready to play, the parent is right there with the child in this strong emotional attunement. In therapy, the therapist has a similarly intense and personal focus on, and engagement with, the child. The goal is to make the child feel seen and noticed. The therapist can use fun or silly activities, like the games we play with babies. The activities have no specific purpose; the point is to be together while paying close attention to each other's responses. This usually gives rise to moments of joint attention and pleasure. Engagement also gives an older child a sense of being seen and of being unique, accepted, and connected. Engaging moments expand positive affect. They are the basis for feeling alive together with someone else.

It is essential for parents to learn to engage more with their child, and the role of the therapist is to support the parents in this process, a topic that we return to in Chapter Eleven. This learning process is especially important for parents who have difficulty achieving synchronicity with their child, either because their temperaments do not match, or because an adopted or fostered child has developed a personality that the parent has difficulty understanding or accepting.

Play is a key form of engagement, and it is typical behaviour in most young animals. The more intelligent a species is, the more the young engage in play. Play involves rehearsing reactions and moves that the young will use when they are adults, but that is only part of the story. In fact, play for the sake of play seems to be an important aspect of life for young mammals. For example, Panksepp (1998; Panksepp & Biven, 2012) explains that play is important both for individual brain development and for the development of social bonds, especially in social species, such as humans. Rough-and-tumble play, one the most common forms of play in young animals, boosts growth factors in the brain that promote cognitive development. Furthermore, all interactive play increases the level of hormones that are necessary for our ability to enjoy interacting with others, especially oxytocin and endorphin. The pleasure of play is an antidote to depression: play and depression are mutually exclusive.

In Theraplay, play and joy are seen as goals in their own right. The focus here is not on symbolic play; everything is concrete, and the play materials are everyday objects that are found in most homes. For example, a cotton ball can be used for gentle touching, it can be blown from hand to hand, or it can be used in a game of football where the players "kick" the cotton ball with their fingers, or in a game where the players face each other on the floor, defining a field with their hands. The cotton ball can be blown back and forth on a sheet of paper or thrown as a volleyball between cupped hands while the players face each other, sitting or standing. Play should be an enjoyable activity; in fact, it can be defined as a physical activity that has joy as its only purpose. Having fun is the hallmark of mental health in a child, and, in most forms of psychotherapy with children, play is an essential element. Also, for the therapist, it marks a genuine connection with the child. Showing the child that one enjoys his or her company, and that the child is someone that it is fun to spend time with helps strengthen the child's sense of self-esteem and self-worth.

At the conference, Jukka Mäkelä explained that the basic idea in much child therapy is to use play as a basic rhythm, the going-on-being of therapy. There are many forms of therapy that use play, but Theraplay contains some unusual elements that do not come from traditional child therapy, springing, rather, from aspects of adequate parenting (what Winnicott calls "good-enough" parenting) or a playful way of parenting. Theraplay uses early interaction play, such as peek-a-boo, as well as later developing rough-and-tumble play, as described by Panksepp (Panksepp, 1998; Panksepp & Biven, 2012), among others. Theraplay also contains elements of mentalization work, but that is done with the parent, not the child. To support the parents' ability to enjoy and engage with their child, the therapist reflects on the child's special character together with the parents: "Who is this child?" They also reflect on and highlight the child's special strengths and abilities, as well as the parents' own experiences in the situation here and now, as they see or experience their child in new ways.

Jukka Mäkelä also mentioned that, in primates, young and adolescent males enjoy playing with younger animals, and the younger the young animal is, the more likely the older animal is to let the young animal win. Similarly, in humans, when an adult rough-houses with a young child, the child always wins. As the child grows older, the child begins to lose more often. Thus, for example, a game where the child attempts to push the adult over is a good way of regulating strength. With some children, it is helpful when the adult puts up strong resistance, yet still eventually allows the child to win. As described in the video clip in Chapter Four, Theraplay uses activities such as thumb-wrestling, pushing games with arms and legs, and fencing with insulation foam tubes. The adult lets the child win and falls over with exaggerated drama, lots of noise, arms and legs flailing in the air. This is a quick way of engaging the child, arousing excitement and laughter and involving the entire body. It is a great opportunity for engaging with a high arousal level, and it can also be used to practise the child's prefrontal impulse control through the ability to stop in an instant in the middle of the joy-filled activity.

In relation to developmental psychopathology, shared joy is the best antidote to continuing depression. It is, for example, very difficult to feel anxiety while playing, just as it is difficult to be depressive and playful at the same. Thus, as described by Panksepp (Panksepp, 1998; Panksepp & Biven, 2012), rough-and-tumble play benefits self-regulation and, hence, also many aspects of psychological development, including the development of executive functions. Panksepp points out that while we do not need the neocortex to play (in fact, it typically inhibits play behaviour), rough-and-tumble play generates brain growth factors that benefit neocortical development. In that sense, play promotes the development of the neocortex, which, in turn, inhibits play. Play-fighting is a hugely important aspect of being a mammal. We learn to control and regulate aggression by play-fighting, and shared laughter is one of the cornerstones of psychological well-being. When we speak of attunement in emotional communication, we often think of calm, sensitive moments, eye contact and shared relaxation, but shared laughter is an equally important attunement experience.

Eia Asen described that he also uses play to promote mentalization; for example, he lets children try to listen in on their parents' minds or thoughts with a stethoscope. This occurs in a play context where the children know that they are merely pretending to be able to "hear" the parents' or their own thoughts through the stethoscope. It is a helpful technique for encouraging children to mentalize themselves or someone else without using the specific terms. He also finds this "game" quite effective in couples therapy: for example, when asking the man to place the stethoscope on the woman's head—"What's going on in there? Amazing!" Eia Asen mentioned a body therapy method that was developed in the 1970s by the Norwegian therapist, Gerda Boyesen, called psychoperistalsis. Boyesen believed that our insides talk to us all the time and therefore put a stethoscope to the body, amplifying the output via a loudspeaker, to hear the body's ongoing responses, for example, in the gurgling of the bowels, etc., even in people with completely normal functioning.

Changes in arousal cause the visceral activity to increase or decrease, which can then be addressed by means of biofeedback methods. It is also possible to use various massage or relaxation techniques, or guided visualisation to reduce the activity of the internal organs, which is a fun activity, especially for boys.

## Joy

Haldor Øvreeide discussed why children smile, and what purpose this non-specific capacity serves. When he sees the smile in his therapy room, or in his supervision of infants on video, he perceives it as the child's way of activating positive emotions or affect in the carers.

It is an important means for the child not only to find the carer, but to find the carer in a state of positive affect in preparation for the interaction. Øvreeide defines it as a present moment when we smile at someone and, thus, hand our affect to the other. This kindles a spark: "When you smile at me, it helps me." He views the child's smile as a crucial aspect of the development process and describes how fatal it can be if someone fails to develop the smile as part of their life. He mentioned one client of his who is unable to smile, and who remains very detached. Somehow, the smile just never entered his life.

Haldor Øvreeide then reminded us of the video recording of Ane Kristine, where she greeted her father with a smile when he entered. Children smile in order to trigger good feelings in the parent; this is not to say, however, that it is the child's responsibility to provide care for their parents, which is something that occurs in very dysfunctional relationships. When the child smiles at her father, she reaffirms their relationship. In relation to this discussion, Jukka Mäkelä responded that children do this for their own sake: Smiling at the parents in a sense lets the parents know that "I need you in order to survive."

Haldor Øvreeide reflected on Jukka Mäkelä's point about the importance of providing the child with a sense of normalcy, for example, by counting fingers and toes and noting that the child has five fingers on each hand. But he also observed how Mäkelä sometimes jokes with the child, saying, "Hey, I found six fingers! We'll have to count again," which intensifies the emotional charge of the situation while drawing attention to a normal feature. It seems that emotions have to reach a certain level of intensity to engage with the more emotional parts of the brain. Jukka Mäkelä agreed that this was a good point, and added that it helps explain why he puts so much energy into creating strong emotions. Haldor Øvreeide explained that essentially he copies good mothers and, perhaps even more, good fathers. For example, when Øvreeide's son had his first child, the father supported the child so that she could stand upright in his two hands and carried her around like that, an experience that the infant girl enjoyed tremendously.

As Haldor Øvreeide pointed out, therapy should not only be fun for the therapist; it should also be a fun and enjoyable experience for the child. Jukka Mäkelä said that he is often asked whether it is all right if only the therapist appears to be having fun, and, of course, this is not all right. After all, therapy is not carried out for the benefit of the therapist. But it *is* all right for the therapist to have fun and enjoy spending time with the child, seeing the child express him/herself and show his or her presence and capacity, as Akil did, for example, when he played the violin with Eia Asen.

## Letting good things happen

At the conference, Jukka Mäkelä pointed out that a therapist should focus on goodness and success. The development of limbic circuits is fuelled by an intense focus on these two things. Many of the children who go into therapy are children who have experienced severe neglect, abuse, or physical trauma. They are children who do not feel that they are all right. Their body is not all right, they are not all right socially and emotionally, and they cannot do the things that adults want them to be able to do. It is not enough to say to the child, "You are a good child," just as it is not enough to tell the parents, "You are good parents." They have to discover it for themselves, based on a true moment, as did the mother in Peter Levine's clip from the session with little Simon. Here, the mother discovered that she was a good-enough mother when the child moulded with her. Children and parents have a moment of discovery when the therapist can point to one small aspect of what is happening and say, "That is good", as when the child pushed Levine's finger put of the way, and he responded, "That's OK, that's fine." That moment enables authenticity.

It is always possible to tell a child "You are beautiful, you are clever, you are good, you are strong," provided one focuses on sufficiently small moments. Jukka Mäkelä has seen cynical foster parents who say, "That will only make him proud, he will become a narcissist if you say nice things about him." But, he asks, what happens if no one ever says anything nice about the child? The foster parents might say, "How can you say that he is such a special child; isn't everyone?" And yes, Mäkelä replies, everyone is, but no one is special unless they are special, unique, and exceptional in someone else's eyes, even if it is just for that one moment where the focus is on what is happening right here and now. Therefore, the therapist must move past the shame and past the traumatic rejection of engagement. The focus should be on that one moment, on the here and now, and on providing clear, positive feedback to the child about this particular moment.

That makes it possible to share pride in mastery and to share the joy of play, feelings that are more or less synonymous with mental health. When the therapist sees something good occur in the session, he or she should make sure that the child and the parents know that the therapist has noticed it, and that it is all right. Intense positive feedback should be one of the common elements of therapy.

## Challenge and surprise

In the relationship between carer and infant, the carer often challenges the child to take small, developmentally appropriate risks and helps the child master tense experiences. Later, the carer supports the child's explorative behaviour, encourages the child to try new activities, and promotes his or her perceived competence. For example, a mother can have the infant "walk" on her lap, or a father can lift his infant high in the air: "You're flying!" When the carer supports the child's development and rejoices in the development of mastery, the child builds confidence in his or her own capacity to learn, handle challenges, and have realistic self-expectations. The message is clear: "You are capable of developing and of making a positive difference in the world."

In a therapy context, challenges are also used to support and promote the child's sense of competence. In Theraplay, for example, activities are designed to lead to success for the child and take place in a playful partnership with the adult. For example, the therapist might help a four-year-old balance on a stack of pillows and leap into the therapist's arms at the count of three. That experience encourages the child to experiment with new activities and builds a sense of competence and confidence. Challenges are part of all children's need to experience development, mastery, and competence. It is fine if the activities are somewhat difficult and require co-operation, but the adult should always choose activities that the child can master, perhaps with a little assistance. The goal is to present the child with activities that challenge his or her current level of development and to make sure that the child experiences success and has a positive experience. The principle of age-appropriate challenges was clearly at play in several of the therapy clips we saw at the conference: for example, in Peter Levine's challenge to Simon when he shook his finger in front of the boy's face, and Simon firmly pushed his hand away. We also saw it in Eia Asen's game with Akil about taking turns at sitting alone in the therapy room. Succeeding in something that is somewhat difficult helps the child grow and develop within his or her zone of proximal development. This principle is applied to ensure that everyone has a positive experience and feels safe and secure, but it can also be used to overcome resistance. Challenges can be used in an attempt to draw the child into an involvement with the therapist. If the therapist suggests an activity that proves to be beyond the child's current capability, the therapist must quickly take responsibility for the failure: "You know what, that was really, really hard! That was hard, let's try something else."

## The therapist as advocate

Eia Asen pointed to another good and important non-specific factor in therapy, which is to have the courage to act as an advocate for the client, when this is appropriate. Much of the work that takes place in the Marlborough Family Service involves cases where there is a clear priority on protecting the child, for example, from emotional abuse from the parents. This protection must always take precedence for a child or family therapist, while therapy must come second. If the therapist feels that a parent is being emotionally abusive to a child in a session, the therapist has to act as the child's advocate and make sure that the child's voice is heard.

Sometimes, a therapist might have to challenge or defy the parents or the authorities if he or she feels that their decisions run counter to the child's developmental needs. Haldor Øvreeide emphasised that this might be necessary, even if one risks becoming moralistic. It is especially important to ensure that the child does not get caught in the middle between the authorities/parents and the "moralistic advocate". Øvreeide pointed out that a truly moral stance could involve intrusion into others' domains, but that working with children also requires exploring the ethical aspects of the relationships and analysing the situation from a moral position and as a power issue. The therapist has a choice to make. For example, it can be very challenging to ask a mother, while her child is present, "What have you told your son?" Here, the therapist puts the mother into a moral position by pointing out her role as carer. Taking responsibility is part of the carer's role.

Thus, Haldor Øvreeide emphasises the importance of being aware of the power issues at play in cases that involve children.

In Haldor Øvreeide's therapy clip with Olaf, for example, the stepfather had been banned from contacting his son and the mother after a fight with the mother. Olaf missed his stepfather, and in the session Øvreeide called the stepfather on the telephone while the boy and his mother were present. Peter Levine called this handling "masterful" and commented that this decision to include the step-father was a courageous decision. In that sort of situation there are many choices available to a therapist, and many might choose to say, "We won't deal with this," and then go back to talking and drawing with the child. Haldor Øvreeide commented that the thera-pist has to know that he or she cannot control the outcome. In this case, there was a good response from the father that the process could build on, but the response could also have been, "Go to hell!" That would then also have been part of Olaf's reality. Jukka Mäkelä pointed out that it takes courage to act as Øvreeide did, because that negative response would also have given the therapist "hell", as he would have had to manage a disastrous position. However, Mäkelä was convinced that this situation, too, would have been managed well, because Øvreeide was aware of the risk and prepared to take on the challenge.

Haldor Øvreeide discussed how the child's therapist is also the child's advocate. There is, for example, a clear point in the incident above that concerns the child's *right* to love his father. This right should be supported, not merely on an abstract level, but in concrete terms. In Øvreeide's therapy with Olaf, the support was quite con-crete, not only with regard to the phone call, but also in the form of the drawing and the envelope, since writing this letter to dad also reduced the unnecessary use of power by the authorities. Here, Peter Levine reflected on one of the PowerPoint slides, in which culture was a triadic element. This is the issue when the therapist must respond to the fact that the child's reality is being challenged by something that does not seem right, whether it is pressure from the mother or from the culture. In this case, the otherwise adequate response by child services included restrictions that were too tight and rendered the family passive. In a sense, the mother was aware that Øvreeide, as a therapist, did not have permission to call the father, and that it was a transgression. The role as advocate involves insisting on the child's rights and making sure that the child is heard. It is a key aspect of any child therapy to amplify the voice of the child.

In the discussion, we pointed out another aspect of advocacy in Haldor Øvreeide's session with Olaf. In the video clip, Olaf had the problem that his mother had collapsed mentally and appeared dissociated. This problem seemed to resolve itself gradually, in part as a result of Øvreeide's advocacy. Another reason it is resolved is that, in his role as advocate and by caring for Olaf and his relationship with the father, Øvreeide not only brought the care for Olaf into the picture but the care for everyone's hearts. Furthermore, Olaf was differentiated from the mother, because her heart was broken, while Olaf's heart was not. This enabled Øvreeide to provide care for the mother, too. She was brought a few steps closer to being able to rebuild herself, which was a precondition for Olaf's improvement. In that sense, the therapist has to act as an advocate, if at all possible, in a way that invites the parent to join in and become an advocate, too. Øvreeide added that, in his assessment, the mother's "defrosting" from her dissociated state was brought about by Olaf's responses to him. On a cautionary note, Peter Levine pointed out the need to consider whether this particular exchange could form a developing pattern that might cause problems for Olaf later, causing a tendency for him to become enmeshed in situations where it is his responsibility to try to bring a more depressed person back to life and feeling deflated if he fails.

## The courage to take a risk

Psychotherapy is about daring and taking risks, which, of course, takes a wide variety of forms. Jukka Mäkelä commented on one example of risk-taking in Haldor Øvreeide's clip from *Skodsborg Observations- og Behandlingshjem*, where an infant girl met her future foster mother (see Chapter Eight). In the clip, the child's familiar carer supported the child in exploring the initiatives of this new adult and helped the two create a new relationship from scratch. The new element was the relationship between the two, but it was created by three persons together: the familiar carer, the infant, and the future foster mother. The future foster mother's contributions were excellent. For example, when she reached out and touched the child's nose, she saw that it was a little too much for the child. When the child with-drew, she then asked the child to point to her (the foster mother's) nose, and the contact was re-established. Haldor Øvreeide commen-ted that in order to reach a child, it is sometimes necessary to dare to overstep the child's boundaries a little bit. The therapist should not intrude, but in order to explore the child one has to overstep the boundary slightly. In this exploration, however, it is essential to respect and register the child's responses.

As Jukka Mäkelä commented, risk-taking is an important non-specific factor. The four therapists agreed that therapy without risk-taking is boring; in fact, therapy without risk-taking probably is not even therapy. Mäkelä referred to the clip where Akil and Eia Asen discussed age and truth, which they did beautifully from symmetrical positions, where Asen did not degrade Akil, but challenged his think-ing. It was a beautiful example of being with the child while pushing the child forward without ever losing respect for the child in the relationship.

In this discussion, we focused on Eia Asen's work. In the clips presented by the other three therapists, the approach to change had been "feminine" or *yin*: a soft, gradual development. Asen's approach was a more "masculine", direct, a *yang* approach to change driven by sudden, dramatic shifts. In relation to the sharp *yang* intervention, we argued that it is probably necessary to observe the interaction for a little while first. The therapist cannot carry out the sharp, dramatic approach in the first second of the interaction, while it is possible to carry out a gentle *yin* contact initiative pretty much from the first moment. When performing a *yang* intervention, one needs to know more before acting. Eia Asen clearly took an initial risk, and that made his approach look very different from the other therapists'. How-ever, we knew all four therapists well enough to know that they all take chances. They all know how to use both *yin* and *yang* approaches, and they include both these approaches in their repertoire. All the sessions we saw at the conference involved risk-taking in either a *yin* or a *yang* approach. There is room and a need for both *yin* and *yang* interventions.

Moments of surprise can be a key element in changing patterns that have emerged and become entrenched as a result of relational disturbances. For example, Jukka Mäkelä commented that when Eia Asen listened to Akil's stomach, this was a moment of change for the boy. Akil discovered that Asen was a crazy guy, and children love crazy guys! There are many ways of being alive, and Asen's approach was a good example of the masculine form that many boys like. It was extremely *yang* with a focus on having fun. However, Asen also followed Akil and entered into important shared experiences, for example, by playing the violin with him. Here, Asen used his strengths, which is what we have to do when we are thrown into various types of interactions and want to follow a child. Asen commented that he saw a similar kind of risk-taking and element of surprise when Haldor Øvreeide decided to take charge and phone the father. Asen commented that Øvreeide would not have made that call unless he felt that there were sufficient resources in the room. Øvreeide confirmed that he knew the mother's personal resources from earlier interactions. He was, of course, also familiar with his own resources and with children's strengths in general—strengths that he mentioned he is constantly impressed by.

Haldor Øvreeide further observed that while they all—Peter Levine, Jukka Mäkelä, Eia Asen. and he—take calculated risks, they are also all quite experienced and have reason to believe that they know what they are doing—more or less. Therapists can never be certain of the outcome, but they can trust that they are ready to pick up the pieces and handle the responses. However, this can be dangerous for younger, less experienced therapists. Therapists have to take calculated risks, but less experienced therapists should not take the sort of risks that he took when he phoned Olaf's father, or the sort of risk that Eia Asen took when he intervened so forcefully in the relationship between Akil and his mother; that takes experience. None the less, Haldor Øvreeide agreed that everyone has to follow his or her own process, and this includes taking calculated risks. As we summarised, it takes experience to assess these relevant risks, and with some clients this type of intervention is not possible. It is also not possible in very brief therapy processes, because the therapist is not around afterwards to follow up on the dramatic encounter. This leads back to the essential nature of psychotherapy. It has to be about psychological development. Psychotherapy should be seen as a developmental process or a developmental interaction. Risk-taking is a key developmental aspect, and constructing oneself through another's gaze and emotionally charged words is a crucial aspect of this development.

## The art of breaking traumatic patterns

Peter Levine mentioned that it can be difficult to break maladaptive patterns in traumas, and that therapy involves understanding the meaning of the deep-seated patterns of self-protection. There are many examples in nature that demonstrate the survival benefits of the freeze response, for example, although it has an incredibly destructive power when it turns chronic. In relation to this discussion, Levine showed a video clip of a cheetah chasing an impala. The cheetah is racing at 100 km an hour, so fast, in fact, that the film is blurred, and we see clips of the cubs that the cheetah needs to feed. After the cheetah has caught her prey, we see a hyena. The hyena knows that the cheetah is exhausted after the sprint, which has drained the predator of energy. The hyena grabs the seemingly lifeless impala, but then steps away for a second—and the impala leaps up and escapes. Levine sees the freeze response as a key aspect of our adaptive evolutionary history. In therapy work with adults, this understanding can often make a big difference. Rather than seeing themselves as weak and passive because they froze in a traumatic situation, the clients can learn to see the response as part of their biological underpinning. Humans have an innate predisposition to approach certain things, such as fresh fruit, and avoid certain others, such as snakes, Resolving a trauma does not mean erasing it; it means releasing the person's potential and capacity for resilience and regulation in many different types of situations. In this, we are not so different from other mammals. Levine described a film clip where a lion had chased down three cheetah cubs that escaped into a tree where they were safe. After waiting here until the lion had gone, they climbed down and then took turns playing the lion, chasing the other two. They kept rehearsing this until they had become as fast as they could. Among all mammals, it is a well-known strategy to learn from experience by reliving and rehearsing events through play.

Peter Levine referred to the girl Susie in his therapy clip, and mentioned that she had a very accurate perception of what had happened. In the clip, we saw her go through the constriction of reliving her younger brother's near-drowning accident. Levine compared the experience to walking along a path, enjoying the scenery of nature—and suddenly seeing a rattlesnake in front of one's feet on the path. One's full attention immediately turns to the snake, and one has no awareness of anything else—trees, leaves, flowers, the little stream—as one slowly backs away to a safe distance. At that point, one opens up to take in the perception of the surroundings again in a shift away from narrow, trauma-based survival-based perception to normal, "soft" perception. This transition is often associated with exuberant displays of joy. Levine mentioned a video recording of a rabbit that escapes after being chased by coyotes. After escaping, the rabbit leapt high into the air in pure exuberance, in a behaviour called pronking, which is often observed in prey animals that get away. Ethologists are unsure about the purpose of this behaviour since it actually slows the animal down, although it might help it leap over a low bush or a similar obstacle. Levine interpreted it as a form of celebration: "Hey! I'm alive!"

To understand what happens in near-fatal events and in the traumas they can produce, Peter Levine pointed to the need to understand the deep-seated structures in our autonomic nervous system. The social engagement system, which evolved in mammals and is particularly powerful in primates, for example, involves a great deal of eye contact between mothers and infants. The fight-or-flight response is characteristic of reptiles, and the shut-down system goes back to the cartilaginous fish and deep-sea creatures, and these systems can become locked. It is particularly dramatic if the shut-down system is locked, because its purpose is to enable us to "play dead", to shut down our metabolism. Many clients who present with symptoms where they are less active, for example, depression, shut-down, and fatigue, are, in fact, stuck in the shut-down response, unlike the impala, which was able to come out of the response again and get away. The reason that these clients have not fully come out of their response is that the reopening process produces sensations that are frightening: for example, sympathetic sensations such as aggression and rage. The therapist, therefore, has to help the client or the child relive these sensations in a limited, contained, and socially engaged way. The social engagement system plays a very powerful role in modulating the sympathetic arousal system. Therefore, when someone has lived through a traumatic event, it is important to have a calm person present who can hold their hand, another human being who is able to connect.

Peter Levine bases this understanding on a neurological analysis. He describes how the lower part of the brainstem connects to all the internal organs, especially below the diaphragm, and affects both our lungs and our heart. The vagus nerve emerges from the brainstem and is one of the twelve cranial nerves. It is the largest nerve in the human body and reaches into our digestive system, connecting the brainstem to all the visceral organs. As 80–90% of this nerve is afferent, it conveys information *from* the gut *to* the brain. Some forms of body therapy, therefore, focus on altering the proprioceptive impulses to the brainstem by touching the client's back in certain ways in order to change this feedback and allow the person to escape from the shut-down state and return to life. This approach has proved effective, for example, with children who have digestive problems and problems with bedwetting. It lets the therapist come in *underneath the radar*, underneath the words, underneath the level of symbols and thoughts.

## Rhythms and the need for repetitiveness in the intersubjective context

In the theoretical section of their presentations, all four therapists emphasised the importance of repetitiveness on the various levels of neural organisation. Peter Levine focused on autonomic pendulation and repetition as means of building resilience when traumatic experiences are the topic of mutual physical play. Haldor Øvreeide described and demonstrated the trust that is built when the therapist repeats the child's statements and, thus, confirms and anchors the prefrontal level in the intersubjective exchange, while Eia Asen used his mentalizing questions to demonstrate the use of repetition as a means of generating a sense of trust and security in the more complex intersubjective context of the brain's second wave of development: for example, by making a game out of sitting alone in the therapy room and by playing the violin with Akil.

Jukka Mäkelä focused on generating development in the "limbic compass" and pointed to the psychophysical facilitation of experiences as one of the basic elements. Mäkelä described how there is always a continuum of experiences that are repeated in the going-on-being of the session, with frequent transitions of different sorts between early interaction or rough-and-tumble play that begin with a simple coming-together activity, then a check-up of the child's special features, for example, eye colour, beauty spots, etc., then activities with increasing and decreasing degrees of intensity. Beginnings and endings are important means of bringing the child into something that is new to him or her. Therefore, there has to be a calming phase and a settling in, with relaxation in mutual contact, in addition to the active play sequences. Social engagement and relaxation are a tremendous capacity to develop for a child who has never been able to do that, as with most of the children that Mäkelä has worked with, who have been fostered after serious abuse or neglect.

## The zone of proximal development

As discussed in Chapter Two, all development takes place in the zone of proximal development, that is, in the areas that the child needs to be able to grow into. Jukka Mäkelä described that being with the child in the zone of proximal development offers an opportunity to activate neural circuitry for the relevant experiences. However, the adult has to guess about the needs of the child and about where the zone of proximal development is. Therapists often work with children who are not following a typical course of development—if they were, they would not be in therapy. The therapist, therefore, has to somehow "cast a net and see whether this net gathers any fish," as Mäkelä put it. If it does not, we cast another net and begin to pull it in, exploring what might help this particular child. Casting the net is the first step. The most important factor, when we begin to pull in the net, is to notice whether there are any fish in it. This means that we notice the child's reactions and consider what they can tell us about the accuracy of our intervention. The adult should not wait for the child to take the initiative, but when the child does take the initiative or react to what the adult does, we have to be ready to grasp it and use it to build the next moment.

The discussion about the zone of proximal development prompted a question from the audience: based on Paul McLean's hierarchical model of the brain, is it possible to affect and reorganise the limbic structures by means of non-specific emotional exchanges in mentalizing dialogues? Jukka Mäkelä felt that this would be possible if there was an area where it was possible to create a dialogue in an attuned relationship. If the mentalizing dialogues are not an area where the child or the parents are prepared to work, the answer would be no. In that case, the situation calls for a stronger intervention, as in Eia Asen's video clip with Akil, where the therapist conveys a message of, "I know that you will both survive even though I am separating you. I can keep you safe, even though you are terrified of dying." As Peter Levine pointed out, the mother was encircling Akil completely, and they needed a strong person to step in and say, "No! This is enough, there are boundaries, you have to begin to separate and become your own being, your own individuated self." We commented that as long as there is interaction among the three hierarchical structures of the brain, an intervention on any of the three levels will also affect the other two levels. If, however, a person is temporarily locked into a traumatic dissociated state, or has suffered early deprivation, there will be very little emotional capacity. In that case, an intervention that relies on a mentalizing approach will have little effect, because the emotional underpinning that is the foundation for mentalizing skills is missing. Instead, the intervention will have to engage the autonomic and the limbic system in order to make a difference.

Peter Levine said that if the nervous system is stuck in a dissociated state, that state constitutes the zone of proximal development that the therapist must work with. Stephen Porges's polyvagal theory describes three basic autonomic systems. One is the mammalian, the more sophisticated system, which deals with social engagement and contact. The other is the sympathetic–adrenal, the fight-or-flight system. The third system is the shut-down response, which is mediated by the primitive dorsal section of the vagus nerve. To illustrate this theory, Peter Levine showed a film clip of a polar bear that had been chased by a helicopter and shot with a tranquilliser. The clip shows the animal coming out of a state of shock in a process that initially resembled an epileptic seizure. When the clip was shown in slow motion, however, it was possible to see that the bear, now semi-conscious and lying on its side, was making running movements, as it had been before it was shot. Next, the bear had heavy breathing reactions that were similar to Simon's reactions in the therapy clip. Levine explained that after major natural disasters, one often finds children with similar reactions. He briefly mentioned a case of a boy who developed hysterical paralysis after a major earthquake. Once his defensive response was re-established, the paralysis was resolved.

For children, the natural response to traumatic events is to seek safety with the carer, but for some children, unfortunately, the attachment figure is also the source of the threat. An infant or a young child cannot fight or flee; his or her only choice is between collapse and attachment. This produces a type of trauma that stems from the child's need to run toward protection and then finding that protection erratic or sometimes violent or misattuned. This traps the child in a para-doxical relationship. However, as illustrated by the clip with Johnny, trauma occurs even when there is a secure attachment relationship. In 1945, David Levy, a child psychiatrist in New York, worked with children who had been hospitalised. A few had been partially immo-bilised by casts or splints for broken arms or legs. All the children had been confined to a hospital setting, which is not a very pleasant place, especially for children. He found that even with ordinary hospitalisa-tions, children developed symptoms that were analogous to the symp-toms in the soldiers he was also working with, who had returned from the Second World War (Levy, 1945). (Although much has improved in hospitals, there are still problems, and children continue to be traumatised. For example, a child should never go under anaesthesia in a frightened state; instead, the child should always be held by his or her parents and given a sedative before being moved into surgery.)

In the following section we will look at the therapist's temporary impact on the child.

### The therapist as the magical stranger—"Mary Poppins"

For family therapy to generate development in the child, the therapist, as a third party, must understand his or her role as a limited and temporary carer for the child. The therapist's purpose is to facilitate an adaptive interaction between parents and child, helping the parents to understand and meet the child's needs in a responsible way that promotes the child's development. When children have experiences of being seen and having their needs met, they will be clearer and more confident in their interactions with the parents.

In the normal carer–child context, the child sees him/herself reflected in the carer's eyes and actions, and that reflection gives the child a sense of whether he or she is worthy of love. The child shapes his or her self-perception and self-esteem based on the adult's attitude. The child achieves joy-filled arousal by means of accurate arousal regulation, where the arousal level is kept just below the point where it is overwhelming. Experiences that combine joy, interest, curiosity, excitement, and peaceful moments form the basis of a relationship characterised by mutual tenderness. The interaction between parents and infants is full of exciting play, which leads to emotional engagement. Many of the games we traditionally play with young children, such as peek-a-boo, blowing on the child's belly, and give-and-take games, draw the child into interactions with the carer and maintain an optimal arousal level. These activities are stimulating and engaging and create a positive self-image in the child. As a result, the child has an experience of being seen as a separate and appreciated person. The child also learns to communicate, to manage intimacy, and to enjoy interpersonal contact. The message is, "You are not alone in the world. You are amazing and unique to me. You are capable of having good interactions with others." However, not all children have had this experience as a natural aspect of being with their carers. That is where the magical stranger comes in. As many of us will recall, the film *Mary Poppins* deals with two children from a well-to-do family who have everything in life except warm, engaged parents. The children's new nanny, Mary Poppins, give them many exciting experiences, but also manages to draw the parents into this universe and, thus, brings the whole family together before she moves on, disappearing out of their lives.

When a therapist enters the child's life as this magical stranger, the child, as Jukka Mäkelä described at the conference, will experience a quick sequence of novel and unusual situations that activate the child's attachment system. This throws the child into a new relationship. The child usually feels safe in this relationship because the parent has already met with the therapist. It is, therefore, important to ask the parent explain to the child that this is a place where there is a nice man or woman who is going to discover new ways of having more fun. Often, when the therapist first meets the child, he or she will say to the child that the two are going to find ways to "make your life with your father and your mother better." The therapist attempts to convey the idea that it should be good, and it should feel nice to be a child with these parents. The child is thrown into this new relationship with the understanding that the parents endorse it, and then a series of fun and exciting activities begin to occur. In a sense, the child encounters an element of surprise in these moments, where the world is not stable, the way it used to be, and a reorganisation has to take place to enable the child to cope with the situation. In a sense, the relationship that the therapist establishes with a child is not "real". One does not establish a long-term therapeutic relationship or a relationship where the therapist becomes a "real" person in the child's life. The therapist is more like a fairy godmother who enters into the situation and does something, gives the child or the parents a present before leaving them to enjoy their newfound relationship. Often, this is the goal of the therapy, and sometimes the process can be quite brief. For example, Mäkelä only spent eight times thirty minutes with Matias before disappearing out of his life again.

In relation to this concept of the magical stranger, Jukka Mäkelä also reflected on Eia Asen's therapy and his way of using a multi-family context as a variant of the "magical stranger" by identifying concentric circles of people who somehow feel a sense of responsibility for the child. In the multi-family context, the other parents and children are brought into a situation where they are, in a sense, responsible for each other. It is one of our key strengths as humans that we can take responsibility for someone who is not our own offspring, which is also what therapists do. We bring in additional resources in the form of families who might otherwise be seen as families who are in need of help from others. Here, they are given a role where they are seen as being able to offer help, which in itself is tremendously therapeutic. In Jukka Mäkelä's assessment, one of the key aspects of multi-family therapy is this practice of bringing in resources from people who thought that they had no resources. In his very emphatic way of moving the mother away from Akil in the first session, Eia Asen similarly showed her that Akil had resources that she did not think he had. Asen said that it took the mother a year to understand it, but even during the first session, the mother actually laughed when Asen asked her (in reference to Akil's behaviour), "And you fall for it?" This small laughter seemed to express, "On some level, I know that this is not true." So, by asking that question, Eia Asen showed her that she had resources. In a variety of ways, the mother showed that she knew that Asen's playful side was a resource.

As Peter Levine commented, all the therapy clips illustrate the archetype of the magical stranger: the person who comes in, brings magic, and then disappears from the person's life again. It is fascinating to see how much can be achieved in a relationship that is not really part of the daily and ongoing reality of relationship. It is not a transference relationship—it is more like a fairy tale, something "not real". Jukka Mäkelä added that the magical stranger is a person endowed with magical powers. For example, Eia Asen used the word "magic" when he talked about the use of masks as means of disguise and concealment as well as protection, entertainment, and magic. In a sense, the therapist always wears a mask because he or she is a "not-real" person in the child's world. The therapist comes in and then disappears again. The therapist comes in with a purpose, tries to create magic, the magic of change, with whatever means are at his or her disposal. This is not about bringing in a method that produces guaranteed results—it is not the method that brings about the change.

Jukka Mäkelä commented that what was demonstrated at the conference was that there is a magic that begins to unfold when someone is ready to take the risk of using whatever is present in the child, in the parent, and in the relationship and begins to work with it. The novelist Ursula Le Guin has explored the concept of magic, and in her books, the wizard always uses whatever is around. The wizard does not bring in curious things like magical wands, etc., but creates something new out of the earth and the ground, like an alchemist.

As Jukka Mäkelä pointed out, Eia Asen similarly uses whatever comes up, just as Mäkelä uses commonplace items such as cotton balls and soap bubbles. The most important element is whatever the child brings into the relationship. In a sense, the magician's mask is that as therapists, we are ourselves, and at the same time we are not ourselves. Asen replied that he believes that Akil accepted him because he could see that Asen could see him for what he was. He felt that he was real, and that he was seen as a real person with real strengths, despite the crazy things Asen did. He also felt that he was taken seriously as a seven-year-old, probably bright, non-autistic, non-damaged person.

## Summary

In our summary at the conference, we pointed out that all the video clips that had been shown included examples of the therapist in the role as the "magical stranger", someone who possesses a distinct ability to see the actual child and to embrace the asymmetrical responsibility while remaining in a symmetrical relationship. One of the qualities that characterise the magical stranger is that he or she is a person of strength who is able to take this asymmetrical responsibility. At the conference, it was repeatedly demonstrated how it is the therapist's personification of this "magical" potential that enables the child to build his or her identity together with the parents.

As Eia Asen rightly pointed out, all the infants and children in the video clips were amazing. In all the clips, the children shone through as the true superstars, and it was impossible not to think, "Aren't they just amazing!" A therapist who is seized by that feeling has a good basis for engaging fully in the process.

# CHAPTER TEN

# Emotions, words, and mentalization

"If we as therapists cannot use words in a way that links experiences with symbols, we will have words that are not words; they are dead words. And we have societies that are full of dead words. A word without emotion is not a word. It does not connect"

(Haldor Øvreeide)

Interventions in child therapy aim to address certain specific levels in the child's nervous system and, thus, reorganise the child's sensing, feeling, or mentalizing nervous system. Through synchronisation with the child's autonomic nervous system and through limbically attuned contact with the child, the therapist has to "challenge" the child's relational patterns in a supportive relationship in order to develop more adaptive relational strategies. The autonomic and limbic exchanges and the non-verbal dialogue shape a creative process where the child's capacity for engaging in the dialogue can develop, and where the child expresses the communication patterns that have been established through previous experiences. From the age of two years, language plays an important role for the child's ability to convey experiences. Although the child expresses emotions and bodily impulses through play and other behaviour, he or she also uses language to engage in dialogues. The better the child is at articulating experiences through language, the better he or she is able to share nuanced experiences and be met with understanding on a mentalizing level.

Mentalization capacities develop through a relationship that consists of interpersonal processes, and the sense of security that is needed to develop mentalization capacities stems in part from the concrete support provided by the therapist. In this chapter, we examine how non-verbal processes develop into mentalizing dialogues that link the autonomic, limbic, and cognitive levels in what we call mentalization processes.

## The role of RIGs for mentalization

As mentioned in Chapter One, much of our personality lies "hidden" in implicit memory schemes, or RIGs. This knowledge is not immediately accessible to the explicit structures and can only become accessible when the areas in charge of our autobiographic memory are activated. Self-reflection is only possible when we engage in situations where the knowledge that lies hidden in our autobiographic memory is recognised. Empathic attunement from the therapist and the safe and structured context of therapy enables the child to tolerate ever higher levels of arousal, which can gradually make room for more memories and thoughts. The final healing process occurs when the child is able to mentalize the life circumstances that created the difficulties. The integration of implicit and explicit knowledge often occurs through narratives and provides the conditions for psychological development and identity growth. One of our most sublime resources is our intellectual capacity to imagine alternatives and other ways of being, acting, etc. Ideally, these processes should be practised with the child while the parents are present (see Chapter Eleven).

As mentioned in Chapter Four, Theraplay work involves four dimensions: structure, engagement, nurturing, and challenge. All these dimensions are present in the autonomic and limbic compasses, and engagement, not least, involves reaching out to another person. Many child therapy approaches involve reaching out in shared play by means of the voice, that is, verbally, but in Theraplay, the reaching out involves physical closeness, touch, and eye contact. The most important aspect of any kind of therapy is to reach out emotionally, and this requires a continuous interest in what is happening here and now. It is this here-and-now that makes authenticity possible because it offers the therapist a framework for describing what is good and strong in this exact moment instead of falling into the abyss of failures and other negative experiences from the past.

## Meaning is created in a relationship but stored in the individual

As Haldor Øvreeide pointed out repeatedly at the conference, we cannot over-emphasise the importance of co-operative interactions. There is always a meaning-making interaction going on, also on the emotional level. This means that we simply cannot establish relationships or interactions without producing some sort of meaning. When an exchange has taken place, and a sense of meaning has emerged, this meaning is stored in the individual. Thus, the individual meets the next moment or the next situation against the background of the meaning that was created in the relationship. This reminds us that while the process unfolds in the relationship, the new meaning is stored intrapsychically, in the individual. We need to respect and meet the child's or the parents' store of information, regardless of level and content. This meaning-making process is always a cornerstone.

## The language that exists before language

Schore (2003b) has pointed out that the right brain hemisphere plays the lead role in implicit or unconscious activity and spontaneous expressions. The right-brain hemisphere enables a "conversation" between two or more individuals' limbic systems, and this is where the therapeutic alliance arises. When the therapist is in empathic attunement with the child's internal state, the contact is intensified and vitalised. The key is to communicate in resonance and to sense intuitively when a state changes. Transference via the left-brain hemisphere also plays a vital and active role in verbal exchanges and logical reflections on the child's life and in relation to the processing of emotions that come out in the course of therapy. Resonance between left-brain hemispheres takes the form of verbal communication, which is linear and logical. Resonance between right-brain hemispheres involves non-verbal components such as intonation, gestures, and facial expressions. The primary intersubjective relatedness, or limbic resonance, occurs through micro-interactions that cannot be prepared ahead of time, but unfold in a process of improvisation that the carer and child create in the present moment (Stern, 1998a,b, 2004).

The left-brain hemisphere masters abstractions, and language lets us build an autobiographical narrative around the internal representations. These narratives are the left-brain hemisphere's way of understanding the personality structures that emerged preverbally, but this understanding is rarely coherent. Children who have been subjected to maladaptive relational patterns, and who have, therefore, been unable to develop a sufficient degree of integration between their right- and left-brain hemispheres, are especially inclined to build a set of narratives around their life story that appears to be dissociated or separated from their implicit knowledge. It is not the reconstruction and the cognitive understanding of the child's history that develops his or her personality, but, as mentioned earlier, the present moments that arise in a relationship. If the words are not related to the experience, they will lack any connection to the child's implicit relational knowledge (Hart, 2010).

At the conference, Eia Asen pointed to the very important non-specific factor of allowing re-enactments in the therapy room, letting feelings come alive rather than merely talking about them in cognitive terms, but making them come alive and enacting them, as Peter Levine had done, for example, with the acts of falling and holding in the session with Susie and Johnny. That makes it possible to re-engage with the feelings that the children might have had while the traumatic event took place. The ability to allow situations and feelings come to life here and now is a key ingredient of good therapy.

In a comment on Peter Levine's video of his therapy work with little Simon, Jukka Mäkelä mentioned that he has seen psychoanalysts working from Françoise Dolto's concept who speak to infants about very complex issues as if the infant was able to understand what they are saying. He always found this puzzling and said that he has no explanation for this state of shared consciousness where an infant responds to words, except to go back to Ed Tronick's idea about the expanded state of consciousness when the infant is in dyadic contact with the mother or another person. Thus, when Peter Levine spoke to the combined mother–baby consciousness, Simon was aware that there had been people who had touched him in ways that were unpleasant, and he perceived something from Peter Levine's tone of voice, but he also perceived how his mother expressed her awareness, because she actually understood the content of Peter Levine's words. In Jukka Mäkelä's assessment, Ed Tronick has an even better under-standing of the expanded state of consciousness than he has been able to communicate; Jukka Mäkelä was convinced that in Peter Levine's session, Simon was able to understand and reach out in a meaningful way. In that sense, Simon engaged in a dialogue with Peter Levine based on his own movements, Levine's comments, and the mother's understanding. In a sense, the triad created a new reality. Peter Levine replied that he had often wondered whether he was being a complete idiot for speaking to babies like that, but that he believes that some-thing happens when we say the words, because we need the words in order to convey the underlying emotion. He does not believe that the infant actually understands the words, but he is convinced that the child understands the feeling that the words trigger in the adult through some sort of resonance, probably mediated by the mirror neurons.

We commented that the key issue is how to create meaning on different levels, and then how to make the different levels of meaning interact. This relates to both the vertical understanding and meaning making among the levels of mental organisation that are such strong factors in Peter Levine's work and to the horizontal understanding and meaning making that stems from how we speak about what happens. In Peter Levine's work with children and mothers and in his work with adults, it seems that a connection is made to the autonomic system through his in-depth awareness of the tiny autonomic move-ments and reflexes. When he works with a child, he articulates this verbally, which conveys this awareness to the mother and helps her see the movements and reflexes as meaningful. In the context of the parent–child relationship, thus, he takes a triadic approach in order to draw the subcortical levels into awareness. Similarly, when he works with adults, the goal is to help the adult's own prefrontal system to become aware of and grasp the meaning of the subcortical processes. Peter Levine always aims to balance the nervous system, for example, by using rhythms; he also checks whether the social engagement system is activated and also offers psychoeducation. Thus, in a sense, his work addresses resources on all three levels.

Jukka Mäkelä mentioned that he had often wondered about the origins of words and what we use words for. The best guess seems to be that words spring from babbling, and very young infants send signals to the parents, and the parents begin to respond. Perhaps humans have evolved because, from the first days of life, infants build relationships with adults, not only with their mothers. In this process, babbling is needed because it reassures the child that the other person is safe and reliable. If the other person answers, he or she can be trusted. From the very beginning, the first rudiments of words are emotional, and the question is whether one's expressions are met with a reply. If this idea about the origins of language is correct, then words without an emotional tone are merely vocalisations that lack the basic element of language, which is to check that you and I are connected, and that I can trust you, because your response lets me know that you have heard me. In that sense, the verbal exchanges in Eia Asen's video of Akil was definitely language, because they served a purpose and created an emotional contact that gave Akil an opportunity to recreate himself.

### The role of present moments for the development of the mentalization capacity

As Øvreeide (in Hart, 2011) has previously explained, the child needs predictability in relationships as well as moments of mutual acknowledgement that may become increasingly predictable in the dialogue. These shared moments convey an experience from one person to another in a way that enables a gradual move towards growing independence as the child gains experience and receives instructions and acknowledgement from the adult that promote the child's capacity for active mastery. The adult's acknowledgement and guidance of the child's attempts at mastering new areas within the child's zone of proximal development form a basic condition for developing social skills. However, the adult also has to protect the child from tasks and responsibilities that exceed the child's capacity and level of maturity. This requires a minimum of acknowledgement and intersubjective dialogue between the therapist and the child, but also between the parents and the child, as we shall see in the next chapter. In the process of unfolding the child's development potential, both children and adults depend on interactions that involve mutually appreciative circularity.

In relation to the appreciative intersubjective dialogic process, one of the questions from the audience concerned the difference between sharing feelings through laughter as against sharing through language. Jukka Mäkelä replied that as long as there is sharing, he was not convinced that there would be a difference. He said that he is sometimes worried about putting strong feelings of connectedness into words, due to a concern that the words might somehow destroy the experience. Daniel Stern has described how the existential and the verbal self can be far apart and separated by language. When children develop language, they are cut off from the direct contact with their own personal experiences, and life as it is lived becomes separate from life as it is narrated. Based on these concerns, Jukka Mäkelä argues that many experiences are best left non-verbal to retain their sense of magic. It is a matter of bringing vitality into the process, and when emotionality is connected with the words, we achieve mentalization—and true poetry.

In relation to the origins of mentalization processes, Eia Asen added that in marked mirroring—letting the child know that one does not feel like the child but with the child—is not a case of the child mirroring the parent; it is the other way around. In marked mirroring, the parent reflects the child's mental state in a slightly exaggerated way. In a sense, the child is "played back" to him/herself in a slightly different version, and, over time, the child realises or learns that the mirroring reflects his or her own state of mind, because it comes back in a slightly different form. Thus, marked mirroring is the parent's active mirroring of the child's mental state. This is also a way of correcting the child's behaviour. For example, if a child is a messy eater, it has a corrective effect if someone else expresses disapproval through marked mirroring. This aspect is used in the multi-family sessions at the Marlborough Family Service. When the families eat together, they all look more or less the same, so if one child eats in a different way, the other families will look at the child, and the other children might comment. This feels less harsh than when it is the therapist who corrects the child. A multi-family context can be useful and serves as a good context for mentalization. The clients see themselves and their family mirrored in the others and encounter a variety of self-descriptions. Observing something in another family might lead to a raised arousal level, but, due to the distance, the arousal is not so intense that it makes mentalization impossible. Often, parents can observe an interaction that reminds them of interactions in their own family, but seeing the pattern unfold in another family causes less arousal than experiencing it in one's own family.

### From language before language to mentalization processes

As Jukka Mäkelä pointed out, mentalization processes play a crucial role, and he has also trained in mentalization-based therapy and appreciates it highly in many situations. Therapies that deal only with the development of arousal regulation capacities and present moments through implicit emotional processes cannot replace the important role of mentalization processes. To be emotionally credible, however, the mentalization process requires a certain implicit element, an element that strengthens the limbic compass to give it the capacity to switch between various emotional valences, to be in contact, and to be with oneself. Theraplay sessions involve a great deal of reflection where Jukka thinks aloud about what he imagines the child is experiencing, but without requiring the child to say yes or no. Of course, the child is allowed to challenge what is said; for example, he might say to the child, "If I'm wrong, you can say that that's not what you're thinking or experiencing."

In Theraplay, the focus is on the messages and on being quick to achieve emotional attunement. One of the fundamental elements is that the child discovers and perceives him/herself through the emotional effect he or she has on the adult, as reflected in the way the adult is encouraged to act in relation to the child's emotions. The child should experience that the adult sees that "my internal emotional world affects you". For example, Jukka Mäkelä described how his own behaviour changed between his first session with Matias and sessions two and three, because Matias's internal world had changed. In the first session, Matias was initially frightened, almost terrified, and Jukka Mäkelä's emotional presence was overwhelming. Consequently, Jukka Mäkelä proceeded very cautiously to ensure a sense of safety. In subsequent sessions, it was much easier to engage Matias's more active sides, being a strong boy, etc. Jukka Mäkelä emphasises that the child's perceived self-esteem comes from being appreciated as he or she is.

## The role of words

Haldor Øvreeide pointed out that words can also play an important role by providing direction. When parents use words, they direct the child's attention to something that might be important. Words can close an experience down, but they can also expand it by directing attention. Eia Asen commented that there should be room for present moments without words as well as present moments with words. There is a time for moments with laughter, for sad moments, and for moments that involve words. A present moment is an important experience, and perhaps it should be put into words later, maybe a week later or some time later, because it shapes our understanding and our sense of being in the world. There could well be a great session that is not based on words or framed in words at the end, and which does not involve any attempt at reaching a rational understanding. Yet, perhaps a week, two weeks, three weeks later, either the child or others might want to reflect on what that experience did, and that, too, can be important. Jukka Mäkelä agreed, and mentioned that, in his opinion, that was exactly what Matias did when when he returned home, and the foster mother called the following Monday to say how wonderful it had been when Matias had come from school and talked about everything that had happened that day in school. She said that on their way home from the Theraplay session, Matias had said, "That was fun!" He was putting the experience into words, and his understanding was that the experience was meant to be fun, and, in a way, that is true: Mäkelä had intended to give Matias the experience that life can be fun. Eia Asen said that if he were in the same situation, he might then ask, "Why did you think that was fun? What was it that made it fun?" He would want to move it up to the frontal brain to try to make shared sense of it. That might then become a now moment between Matias and his mother. We added that the more limited the mentalization capacity, the greater the emphasis on the experience in the therapy room; the greater the mentalization capacity, the more room for including mentalizing processes. Generally, we are a speaking species, and we all use words every day for all sorts of purposes. The key for therapists is how to bring words into the emergent therapy process in a good way, where experiences are linked to symbols. If they are not linked to experiences, words are dead, without any emotional and, thus, mentalizing content, and in many ways, we live in a society full of "dead" words. As Haldor Øvreeide concluded, a word without emotion is not a word. It does not connect.

One of the participants asked how important the specific words are that the therapist uses and whether it would be possible to use an interpreter in this type of work. Peter Levine replied that in therapy with older children, he has sometimes worked with an interpreter, but since so much of his work takes place in the non-verbal sphere, words are often superfluous. He mentioned working with a child with autism in Zurich. The main goal of the therapy was to help him understand that he had a body, and that all the parts were connected. If the boy became excited, he would instantly fall asleep and, thus, slip out of contact. Peter spoke English with him and felt that having an interpreter might have interfered with the flow. If translation was absolutely necessary, both the mother and the grandmother were present, and they both spoke some English. Peter Levine said that he had recently received an email saying that the boy had now started in a special needs school. In therapy without words, much of the focus is on seeing what is going on beneath the words.

Jukka Mäkelä spoke of his experiences from a therapy process where he used an interpreter in working with the parents, but relied on his own native language of Finnish when he worked with the child and the parents together. The parents and the child did not need to understand much of what was said, as Jukka Mäkelä was able to describe what was going to happen without relying on words. However, he did use an interpreter to prepare the parents before the joint session with the child. Eia Asen said that the Marlborough staff often worked with interpreters, but that they trained the interpreters to work in a way that does not interfere with the process; the interpreters, on the other hand, trained the therapists to speak in way that they could translate properly. When working with an interpreter, it is important to position the therapist directly across from the child and/or the parent and to avoid looking at the interpreter. There are a number of techniques that can be used to help overcome the language barrier.

## *Supporting the child's development of emotional and mentalizing capacities by co-operating with the parents*

In the next chapter, we take a closer look at the importance of including the parents in child therapy. For the child to develop, the parents have to be able to mentalize their child, so, in this section, we look at how the child develops mentalizing processes through the therapist's co-operation with the parents. As Eia Asen pointed out at the conference, the child needs the parents to understand the impact that their actions, feelings, and behaviour have on the child; similarly, the parents need to be aware of how the child's behaviour affects them. In some parents, this capacity is not very highly developed. In recent years, he has worked with Peter Fonagy and others to develop techniques that they think will be able to improve people's awareness of the impact of their own actions or emotions on others, and *vice versa*. Eia Asen saw it as absolutely crucial to include this aspect in the therapy process. In the video clips with Akil, at one point, the mother realised that "my son can read my mind. He is looking at me, and he knows what I'm feeling, and maybe that's not so good." The mentalization process unfolds as Eia Asen reflects with her on what she might do to keep her son from being overwhelmed by her worries, feelings, fears, and anxieties.

Haldor Øvreeide commented on the fact that Eia Asen had discussed Akil with the parents while the boy was in the room, which Haldor Øvreeide called a "behind the sofa" situation, where Akil overheard the parents and the therapist caring about the child. They spoke in a respectful and caring way about how they could best understand Akil. Haldor Øvreeide said that these are important moments in the therapy context for children to feel safe and develop a trusting relationship with their parents where they are not directly engaged, but are able to observe or feel that the parents care for the child emotionally. This is also what the Danish therapists Inger Thormann and Inger Poulsen do in their brand of infant therapy (Thormann & Poulsen, 2013), which is inspired by the French psychoanalyst, Françoise Dolto. They create a situation where they speak to the infant about his or her background history and develop a special emotional atmosphere that appears to have a profound developmental effect on the infant. The video of Eia Asen's therapy with Akil showed a similar process, which established an atmosphere of relevant care. This phenomenon is equally important whether the therapy involves an infant or a much older child. Even if children might not understand exactly what is being said, they are receptive on a level that we can barely grasp the full importance of. Eia Asen confirmed that he also viewed it as important to allow the child to be a listener. When we are placed in a third-person listening position, we hear things differently than when someone addresses us directly; the way we listen is more affective than cognitive. Often, when children appear to be playing with something, they have better ears than if an adult addresses them directly; often there is so much stress, so much focus on them that they shut down.

To support the development of both the child's and the parents' mentalization capacities, Eia Asen's work often includes masks. He quoted Oscar Wilde: "Give him a mask, and he will tell you the truth." Masks can serve many different purposes. They allow us to hide ourselves. They can protect, entertain, and add a touch of magic. They allow us to bare aspects of ourselves that are not normally embraced in our day-to-day lives. They cover up our identity, shielding our true emotions and giving the imagination free rein. Masks invite us to tell a story and can help reveal how others view us from the outside and how we feel on the inside. Eia Asen said that, at the Marlborough Family Service, they use masks more and more. Therapists either buy masks or make masks for specific purposes. The masks serve a variety of purposes; for example, one advantage might be that one's face is no longer available for being "read". Eia Asen described how some children could not bear being cut off from the parent's face and had been compelled to tear the mask off. These children were encouraged to be like Buster Keaton, maintaining a deadpan expression without the mask. When therapy involves masks, the session is recorded to allow the therapists to review the session later and reflect on what is going on inside the child. That allows a lot of speculation, not only in the now moment, but also as something that can be addressed in a subsequent review together with the family.

Eia Asen explained that he sometimes finds that a child's irrational thinking really reflects the parents' irrational thinking. He described an eight-year-old boy who had once been a patient of his. The child had the delusion that there was someone "up there" looking into his head. Afterwards, the mother asked to speak to Eia Asen and told him, "The only reason why I'm here now is I want to check that there are no hidden cameras in this room." Eia Asen assured her that there were no cameras, but she still insisted on inspecting the room carefully. He became interested in the mother's story, and she said that both her brother and her late sister suffered from schizophrenia. When her son was born, she looked at him and wondered, "Is he schizophrenic, or is he not schizophrenic?" So, since he was one week old, this boy had been under close observation from his mother, who was checking for possible signs of schizophrenia.

In the video with Akil, we saw how Eia Asen introduced the globe when he asked Akil to show him where his parents came from. Haldor Øvreeide said that, to him, this was one of the highlights of the therapy process: there is a globe in the room, the child goes over to the globe, Eia Asen picks it up, and together they bring it into shared focus. Eia Asen asked the unasked questions on behalf of the boy, he challenged the parents to share something about their background, which is often taboo, for many reasons. Anyone who is a victim of circumstance is also a victim of shame, and, thus, in many cases, themes that are associated with shame in the parents' mind will also affect the children. In the session, Eia Asen had broken the spell of shame by helping the child ask what Haldor Øvreeide characterised as "the unasked questions". Jukka Mäkelä added that Eia Asen had done it in a fun way by talking about being "the nosy child" and making it all right to be a nosy child. It is all right to ask difficult questions, and so, asking questions without feeling shame offers a way out of the individual patterns of shame that have been stored against a background of family secrets, which are considered taboo.

Inspired by the issue of taboos, Haldor Øvreeide then addressed the very essential issue of what to do when a relationship is past healing. As he pointed out, there are always developmental possibilities for the individual, but development requires a supportive relationship. Some relationships have moved past the point of no return, where they cannot be fixed, and that poses a huge problem for children.

Psychotherapists often wish to repair relationships that are incapable of returning to safe and supportive positions, because the abuse or neglect has been so severe. A key issue is where the point of no return is: when is a relationship so damaged that it cannot be repaired? In Haldor Øvreeide's assessment, this questions touches on a taboo, because it interferes with the parent–child relationship and our social or cultural construction of this relationship. Jukka Mäkelä welcomed Haldor Øvreeide's contribution in raising this point and added that the key question is how we construe understand parenting as a cultural construct, and how human parenting has evolved throughout history. Traditionally, childcare has always been provided by "mothers and others"; mothers have always needed other people's involvement to provide the sort of parenting the child needs. Today, we tend to think that either the parent is good enough, or, if the relationship is no longer sound, the child should have a new set of parents, which means being fostered or adopted. Jukka Mäkelä argued that we need to consider how many "others" the child requires in order to develop. In Jukka Mäkelä's assessment, probably no relationship is really past the point of no return if it is relieved of most of the responsibility of what it could have been. He admitted that this assessment might be idealistic, but he still felt that, in any fragile relationship, there is an element of wanting to be meaningful to the other and a lack of capability to be meaningful in a safe and secure relationship. Those cases would require extensive contributions in the form of foster care and therapy for the parent, and, in that sense, the "others" would become more important than the mother. However, that should not mean giving up on the relationship, because, from the child's point of view, the relationship with the parents never ends.

## Summary

This chapter addressed the role of the development of language and mentalization in the psychotherapy process. The essential point is that meaning is not created by verbal descriptions, but by interactions and, especially, attunement processes in an emotional relationship, which are subsequently stored in the individual as internal, generalised representations, so-called RIGs. Self-narratives and reflection can, therefore, unfold only against the background of a functioning limbic representation formation. Haldor Øvreeide and Jukka Mäkelä pointed out that, in expressing the emotional relationship, verbal communication supports the connection between the limbic and autonomic levels of organisation and verbal consciousness. Used in this way, words convey meaning and coherence for the child. Eia Asen underlined the importance of allowing feelings and situations to arise and come to life in the therapy room, and, based on Levine's therapy with Simon,

Peter Levine and Jukka Mäkelä discussed how words can also be used as meaningful projectors into the child's non-verbal states. The therapist and the parents can use language to achieve a shared understanding of the meaning of narratives, or linguistic meaning. Infants, on the other hand, perceive in ways we probably do not understand, but they capture the preverbal meaning expressed by carers and the resonance that the shared description creates for the adults.

Another aspect of the role of language was discussed in relation to Eia Asen's therapy with Akil and his parents, where he unfolds the role of the therapist in modelling "the nosy child". With his own questions, the therapist supports the child and, indirectly, the parents in initiating a dialogue about questions in the family's history that are "unasked" and often taboo. Eia Asen also pointed out that the reflective questions are a key instrument for inviting mentalizing reflections from parents and children. Language is also used to frame the relationship: for example, in descriptions that support the generational hierarchy and the role of the parents. As a follow-up to present moments, language can also be used to point out the qualities that the child has just demonstrated, thus supporting the child in "recreating him/herself" in his or her own eyes as well as in the eyes of the parents.

# CHAPTER ELEVEN

# Parental involvement

"The child comes into development with an intrinsic motivation for developing, and in order to unfold, this motivation
must be met by relevant responses from carers. However, this
project is embedded in another project, which is a cultural
project. The parents are also coming into the situation with a
cultural project that they bear on their shoulders"

(Haldor Øvreeide)

O
ur culture is constantly changing. Bowlby (1988) noted that,
in previous generations, mothers had been surrounded by
their mothers, teenage sisters, cousins, etc., who were all
involved in raising the children. These helpers not only gave the
mother a chance to take breaks from their role as carers, they also
offered friendship, good advice, and confidence. The child had alternative attachment figures, which took some of the pressure off the
attachment and the relationship between the parents and the child.
Changes in the way we live have made the family system more
vulnerable, and any inadequacies in the parents' carer functions can
severely damage the parent–child relationship, because there is no

family network to take over temporarily if the parents become over-burdened (Hart, 2010). As early as in 1946, when Bowlby began working at the Tavistock Clinic in London, he did therapy with parents and children that included the whole family. Although family therapy was not widely recognised until the 1960s, the first seeds were sown in the 1920s in the USA, when the psychiatrist Harry Stack Sullivan described mental illness as an interpersonal disorder. The anthropologist Gregory Bateson is known especially for laying the philosophical groundwork for the systemic mindset and treatment method, which developed in the 1950s and 1960s. In the 1970s, structural and systemic family therapy developed, and, as described in Chapter Two, it has had a tremendous impact on our understanding of how interpersonal patterns develop into an intrapsychic state.

Whether the therapist chooses to initiate the intervention in the context of the family system in conversations with the whole family, with just the parents, and/or with just the child, the overall focus should be on the whole family system, and the parents should always be included in the treatment context. For example, the intervention might target the parents by addressing their internal representations and parenting behaviour, and the therapist might support the child in developing a more accurate perception of the attachment figures and attuning emotionally with them in order to offer the child alternative and positive relational options. It is important to keep in mind that the intervention should not get in the way of a development of the contact between the child and parents by having the therapist take over the carer's functions.

Psychotherapy with children is not a compensatory solution that is put into place when the carers are unable to provide adequate support for the child. The communication and the relationship between the parents and the child is an important focal point for the therapist's work, regardless of whether the parents are included in the intervention. As far as possible, the primary carers should be supported in engaging in attuned contact and in creating a developmentally supportive dialogue with the child. Based on Winnicott's thesis that an infant can never exist outside a relationship, psychotherapy can only support adaptive development if it involves the primary carers. Without including the things that the carers bring into the relationship and their perception and understanding of the child, it is difficult to achieve any improvement in the parent–child interaction.

As Brazelton and Cramer (1990) have stated, a carer needs to be both selfless and selfish: selfless in being able to see the child's point of view, and selfish in desiring feedback from the child. A carer and a child who are able to engage in synchronised behaviour will develop a shared dialogue. They are able to engage in rhythms with specific rules, and, as they become familiar with each other's abilities to engage in interactions, they can use these rhythms to establish expectations about what maintains the rhythm, and what disrupts it. Autonomy develops from the certainty of knowing one's carers, which implies that they are predictable. Just as child therapy involves focusing on the relationship between the carers and the child, the relationship between the carers and the psychotherapist is also important for changing a maladaptive relationship between the child and the carers. In this context, the therapist should be able to support an adaptive interaction between the child and the carers by promoting trust, relief, and growth through synchronisation. The communication and relationship between the carer and the child form an essential focus for the psychotherapist's efforts, whether the parents are taking part in the conversation or not.

As described in *Neuroaffektiv psykoterapi med børn* (Hart, 2011), family therapy often involves a combination of family conversations and conversations with just the parents and/or the child. For example, conversations with the parents might be necessary if a marital conflict is hampering the child's development, or if there is a troubled field of tension between them. Conversations with the parents alone may also deal with their internal representations and any stressors that do not directly concern the child. For some time, the child might need to discuss his or her difficulties with a neutral person because the child feels insecure about the parents' reaction. It is of little use to the child to take part in therapy with the parents, only to hear them speak about the child and his or her behaviour in negative terms. Instead, if the parents receive an appropriate reward from the child's response, they will develop along with the child. Each new stage in the child's development pushes the parents to adapt, and, step by step, they learn more about themselves and their own development while learning about their child. The strategies that children use to bring their parents out of a non-responsive state show the seriousness of the child's reaction. Reciprocity and the shared achievement of goals through social interactions make up a necessary basis for the development of affective well-being in childhood.

The most efficient therapy for parents who are unhappy about their child's maladaptive behaviour is to help them to work with their child in a sufficiently sensitive way. When they see their child discovering his or her internal organisation, learning to control over-reactions and accepting and responding to social stimuli, the parents can begin to find techniques for stimulating and helping the child overcome his or her difficulties in a way that the therapist might not even have thought of. That is why it is so important to include the parents in the context of family therapy and also, in therapy with the child, to attempt to develop the parents' ability to mentalize the child. As mentioned in the previous chapter, mentalization capacities develop through interpersonal processes in the context of a relation-ship. This principle applies to both children and adults. The parents need to experience themselves as meaningful in the eyes of the thera-pist and as persons who are doing their best. The sense of security that is need for mentalization capacities to develop comes in part from the therapist's specific support for the parents in the therapy process.

## A dyadic process with triadic consequences

If a therapist chooses to engage in child therapy from a family ther-apy perspective, Øvreeide (2001, 2002) and others have pointed out that while the dialogue between a therapist and a child is dyadic in process, its consequences are triadic. Øvreeide's point is that engaging in a therapy process with a child gives the child an opportunity to be seen and contained with his or her difficulties, but is also gives the parents an opportunity to see their child in a new light. The therapist attempts to establish the attunement and dialogue with the child that the parents failed to establish, as the child's difficulties often stem from the parents' failure to attune with the child's needs and prob-lems. When the child is unable to attune with his or her carers in rela-tion to specific experiences or mental images, the child is isolated. When that is the case, for the sake of his or her identity development, the child needs help with verbalising his or her experiences as well as the experience of being seen by another person.

As Øvreeide (2001) explains, it is the therapist's task to see and affirm the suffering that the child has experienced and the competence that he or she expresses; another task for the therapist is to make the child's needs and competences visible to significant others. The next stage is to register, acknowledge, and, perhaps, to challenge the reactions of both the child and the parents to what happens and to support more adaptive reactions from the parents in relation to the needs and states that are present in the child. Øvreeide mentions that the therapist's dialogues with the dependent person (the child) and the person in charge (the parent) should always contain both affirmative and challenging elements. In the therapy context, the establishment of a secure base is a crucial condition for any successful intervention, and the parents need to know that the therapist is not just there for the child, but also for them, and that the therapist can be trusted.

At the conference, Haldor Øvreeide highlighted the importance of the dyadic nature of human communication; for example, we nod when we listen to someone. He mentioned that if someone in the audience were to nod at him, that would constitute a little exchange between them, and this exchange would continue when he then looked at the person and kept talking; the person might then nod again, and, in that way, the conversation would continue. This communication would unfold in a dyadic relational context while the rest of the audience listened in. Now, if that person had a special place in Haldor Øvreeide's heart, and his wife were sitting next to him, she would pay very close attention indeed to what was unfolding in this dyadic interaction. Thus, in a sense, the dyadic communication always plays out in a triadic, multi-relational structure or context. We cannot communicate with someone without considering whether others might take an interest in what is going on inside the dyad. That is why Haldor Øvreeide finds it so important to bring the parents into his working process with the children.

Dialogues are a sort of intersubjective shared experience of the world, and in the dialogue we begin to be able to appreciate and acknowledge the other's mental state. The video with Ane Kristine showed how the mother and the little girl entered into an intersubjective interaction in relation to the environment. In this situation, the father and Ane Kristine had not yet arrived at a place where he was able to acknowledge her mental state. When the intersubjective capacity emerges, the parents' resources also unfold in the situation. The shared resources are accumulated in the situation, there is support and caring, the child receives new information, and there is attachment and loyalty. Thus, the process has multiple end products.

## Therapeutic examples of work within a
## dyadic process with triadic consequences

As an example of child therapy processes that let the child be seen and contained with his or her difficulties, and which offer the parents an opportunity to see the child in a new light, Eia Asen highlighted a sequence in Peter Levine's therapy with little Simon. He had found it interesting to see how Peter Levine had approached the child and the mother physically, and how he first connected with the mother. He had noticed the rattle and the sensitivity with which Peter Levine then pulled back when he saw that Simon did not want the rattle to connect with him. He had also noticed Peter Levine's tone of voice and his use of the phrase, "You're a spinner," which immediately sparked reso-nance with the mother who answered, "Yes, he's a spinner!" Eia Asen pointed out that this "spinning" helped to connect the three of them; certainly Peter Levine and the mother were now spinning the same theme.

Eia Asen had also found it intriguing to see how Peter Levine mainly addressed the infant and, thus, indirectly, the mother through the child. Because Simon was on his mother's arm, she felt her child, and the child felt his mother's response. In Asen's assessment, that bio-feedback cycle clearly played an important role. He was less sure about how the mother actually fed back her own emotional state to the child. He was interested in Peter Levine's way of positioning himself in relation to the mother and child as an example of the more general considerations in how the therapist should position him/herself physically in relation to the family and the child. He had noticed that, at first, Peter Levine sat next to Simon and his mother, not across from them, which Eia Asen felt was a good choice; when meeting someone for the first time it helps not to sit opposite them, but side by side. Peter Levine commented that when he worked and taught in a Hopi reservation, he had noticed that when people were getting to know each other they never sat face to face; they always sat side by side, and eventually they would make contact. Haldor Øvreeide added that in sessions with children, he always works triadically with the child and the mother, where he constitutes the third party; he also always avoids sitting directly across from the child because he wants to activate the child's agency. Sitting side by side requires the child to be more active, and it requires the therapist to show more active engagement when the two talk or interact, and that enhances the communication; face-to-face interactions are quite demanding and tend to hamper the other's agency. In his assessment, therefore, the issue of power relations also plays a part.

Haldor Øvreeide was curious to know what Peter Levine specifically does to connect with the mothers. He had noticed that Peter Levine used his voice very deliberately, in almost the same way as a mother speaking to her child, but he was curious about what Peter Levine does to elicit the mother's competences during the therapy process. Peter Levine explained that in the session with Simon, he had been watching the mother almost as closely as he had watched the child. Even when he was looking at Simon, he was still aware of what was going on in his peripheral vision, and he knew that if Simon wanted to move towards moulding with the mother, and she was not ready, the process would defeat the purpose of the therapy. He mentioned that he was very fortunate in that he is not working with mothers who have a very disturbed attachment capacity. In the video clips that he used at the conference, the mothers are clearly "good enough", in Winnicott's sense, and he has very limited experience of working with disturbed mothers. In his therapeutic work, he said that he often chooses to work with the mothers first to help them regulate in order to facilitate the subsequent supportive work with the child. Peter Levine mentioned that when he was in practice, 99% of his work was with adults, and that everything he knows about child therapy he has learnt from children, by observing and interacting in play, which has also, in turn, facilitated his work with adults.

Jukka Mäkelä commented that he had noticed how Peter Levine was able to connect with the mother and work with her through the way he spoke to Simon. For example, he had noticed the moment when Peter Levine commented on Simon's pushing him away: Peter Levine had said, "That's OK," and Jukka had noticed how this made the mother relax. When a child opposes an adult, for example by pushing the adult away, the parent will often be anxious, thinking that their child has misbehaved. By saying "That's OK," the therapist reassures her that "This is a good-enough baby, which means that I'm a good-enough mother." She does not need to see the act as an act of rejection. Jukka Mäkelä saw that this initial approval eventually led to Simon pressing his head against the mother's heart after all those months of not being able to relax with her. Thus, an important non-specific factor is how to regulate both the child and the parent at the same time; Peter Levine not only regulated Simon and he not only interacted with the mother, but actively sought to bring the two together and into the same universe. It is important to understand Simon's movements as meaningful in the context of the work that is going on, not only as response to a stranger but as a meaningful statement.

Haldor Øvreeide commented that much of his own therapy work and the work that Peter Levine had presented aimed at helping the mother understand and make sense of the child's actions, which had until then appeared nonsensical to her. That re-establishes her connection with the child and activates natural resources or healing. To understand the child and to be able to make sense of what the child does are crucial factors in the carer–child contact, and if these factors are not in place, the mother is bound to feel that she is failing. Eia Asen brought up the incident where Peter Levine was the one who caught Johnny, as he was rehearsing falling, and the mother was watching. Eia Asen wondered how the mother felt about Peter Levine being the safe person who caught the boy, seeing the children feeling more and more relaxed in falling and being caught, and wondering also if it would be helpful to hand this role over to her. Peter Levine explained that he was monitoring the mother as this was going on, and that he had spoken with her and her husband the night before, and they both seemed pretty secure in themselves. The mother had been an Olympic swimmer and was carrying feelings of guilt for not making the pool child-safe despite her expert knowledge, and Peter Levine felt that if he had tried to involve her it would have defused the energy of the process, and he would not have been able to go for the specific things that he was aiming for because the children's reactions were unfolding so fast. He explained that normally, when he works with a mother, especially in connection with a birth trauma, and he is holding the infant, he moves gradually towards the mother and eventually hands the child over to her. Jukka Mäkelä commented that, in his experience, it is essential to be certain that the parents are able to enter into the situation. It might be helpful to rehearse the situation with the parents first through a role-playing activity. If that has not been possible, then it might not be safe for Johnny, for example, to leap into his mother's arms at that time. Thus, the best approach might be for the therapist to go first and bring in the mother later, after making sure that she has the capacity.

At the conference, Jukka Mäkelä presented a video to demonstrate how he worked in a dyad and then triangulated the parents into the process. The video shows Waqar, a preschool boy, sitting in a beanbag chair. Jukka Mäkelä is stroking his hair, blowing on his hair, and touching his face. Waqar had a little scratch on his forehead, which Jukka Mäkelä attended to. Waqar smiled, and the two had intense eye contact. The boy seemed calm and happy and raised his hand to initiate play. Jukka Mäkelä responded to this initiative, and they began to play a little game with hands and fingers. Later, Waqar climbed up to stand on Jukka Mäkelä's shoulders, laughing and looking proud and excited. Jukka Mäkelä said, "You are really good at this." He then helped Waqar climb back down, and then Waqar pressed his hand against Jukka Mäkelä's hand, and Jukka Mäkelä invited him to ". . . push as hard as you can!" When the boy did this, Jukka Mäkelä fell backwards in an exaggerated fall, and Waqar laughed. Jukka Mäkelä commented, "And you have such a beautiful laugh. Ah, but I see that you can make all sorts of expressions. Can you do this one? Can you be angry? Oh yes, really good. How about . . .? Yes!" At this point, the mother's therapist asked the mother to go into the therapy room, and she was immediately drawn into the play. In the first activity, Waqar had to balance a beanbag on his head, and Jukka Mäkelä instructed him, "When mummy says so, you nod your head, so the beanbag falls down." The mother let Waqar wait a little bit too long, so the bag begins to topple off. Still, he was able to wait, and they had intense eye contact. In this activity, Waqar showed his mother that he had self-control. The most important incident for the mother was when she forgot the special word she had to say to Waqar as a sign that he drop the bag, and Waqar showed that he was able to wait and wait and wait. Eventually, he told her what the word was; she said it to him, and he dropped the bag. This let her know that she was capable of co-regulating with Waqar.

Haldor Øvreeide commented that he found the level of engagement in Jukka Mäkelä's work fascinating, but that he also wondered about the degree of intimacy with the child. He said that he sometimes encounters this issue of intimacy as either a problem or a resource. It can be tricky to handle, although he does think it is important, as Jukka Mäkelä did, to include the parents in the situation and eventually reinstall the intimacy where it belongs: in the family. If that does not happen, the therapist risks ending up as "that nice therapist who left me!" In other words, the relationship is not triangulated—it does not develop into a triadic process.

Jukka Mäkelä explained that he usually includes the parents at a very early stage in the process, especially when the process calls for intimacy. In the video with Matias, the team already knew the foster mother because they had worked with her before in connection with another child. The foster mother was not a very emotional person, so he was concerned as to whether she might be afraid that Matias would reject her, as he had done for years, and, unfortunately, the intervention with Matias would have to be brief. If the family had lived in Helsinki, they could have arranged for more time, but she lived far away in eastern Finland, so they only had two week-long holidays. The team also knew that the boy and the mother would probably have more in common on the more active side of their future relationship. However, establishing intimacy is about establishing a capacity for intimacy and then turning it over to the primary carers as soon as possible. Of course, this could be a problem: for example, if the foster parents have difficulty accepting the intimacy and think that the child's difficulties are inherent in the child and, hence, the child's own problem. It is difficult to work with intimacy if there is no one to whom to transfer it.

### Therapeutic work with parents through the child or working with their parents in their own right

A question from the audience asked what Peter Levine would have done if Simon's mother, too, had been traumatised. Would he have worked with the mother's trauma first, before working with the child, or would he work with them both at the same time? Peter Levine replied that he would have done both, especially if there was a blockage, a resistance to connect with the child. Initially, it would have been possible to address the experience of not being a "good enough" mother that would invariably result if a mother has difficulty connecting with her child. However, when Simon moulded with his mother the way he did, she had the miraculous experience that "This is my new baby!" In a way, it is the infant who takes the initiative; for example, when the parents look at their child and receive a smile in return, it is hard for them not to fall in love with the child. As Jukka

Mäkelä added, it is far more effective to have the child tell the mother what he experiences in her. It is difficult to see how it would be possible to work with the mother's trauma without having the child tell her, physically, that "I accept you." Just as therapy requires bringing vitality into the therapy room, it also requires bringing out the resources, both the mother's and the child's.

Eia Asen mentioned that the Marlborough Family Service does a lot of work with traumatised parents and children, including parents who have been subjected to torture in other countries, and who have a hard time holding the child or the infant in their awareness, because they are so overwhelmed by their own experiences. In his assessment, it is often necessary to begin with the parents and work with their traumas first, before they are able to focus on the child's trauma. He concluded that there is no clear-cut answer, because there are many different contexts, which call for different approaches. Peter Levine agreed, and added that he would not dream of putting the child and the mother together right away if the mother was severely traumatised—it simply would not be an option.

## The therapist as the parents' role model

In addition to working with the parents through the dyadic process, which, as Haldor Øvreeide pointed out, is triadic in consequence, another option is to work with the parents by positioning the therapist as a role model. In Theraplay, for example, there is an explicit understanding with the parents that they are not required to take the lead in the therapy room, whatever the child does; in the therapy room, the therapist is responsible for everything that happens. This means that while any success belongs to the parents and the child, anything that goes wrong is the therapist's responsibility. That relieves both the child and the parents of the pressure of having to be "good" or "clever", and that releases their energy, enabling them to try new things and have fun together. For the child to be free and spontaneous, there has to be an adult who takes the responsibility. Naturally, the responsibility should eventually be transferred to the parents, as one of the key elements of Theraplay is that the adult always carries the responsibility, but initially, they are allowed to lean on the therapist as a role model.

At the conference, Jukka Mäkelä described the very concrete approach to the use of role models in Theraplay. He explained that the parents have their own therapist, who helps them understand what is happening. Parents often ask, "Why is the therapist doing this simple stuff; he's seven years old, after all, why are they counting his toes?" Theraplay always begins with a session just for the parents, because that is the simplest way to explain what is going to happen. The parents are asked to come in, and the therapist does a Theraplay session with them, where they play together. This makes it easier for them to understand what the child is going to experience. After this initial session, the parents come in every fourth session or so, without the child, to reflect and think about what they will be doing with the therapist the following three sessions, and what sort of issues they will be addressing.

At first, the parents observe through a one-way mirror or a monitor. The parents sit with their own therapist, who helps them reflect on what they are seeing, the child's actions and reactions. By observing the child together with their therapist, the parents learn about the importance of being able to receive as well as to give. Fairly quickly, depending on when the parents feel comfortable, they begin to take part in the sessions with the child. Jukka Mäkelä has noticed that many parents do not feel comfortable playing, perhaps because no one played much with them when they were children. Therefore, before the parents are included in the sessions with the child, it is always helpful to show them what to do, how to practise, and how to make the activities safe for the child, so that the child can feel certain that the parent will catch the child in his or her arms, for example, when the child jumps. In the child's final session, the therapists have rehearsed the activities with the parents, so that they are able to take the lead. The idea is for them to pick up ideas from the therapy and work on them at home. Usually at bedtime, they will play a little game where they put on lotion, count toes, or sing to the child, or, perhaps, when the child comes home from school, they set aside a special time just for having fun together, before the child has to do homework, for example. The idea is that both the child and the parents know that they have assignments, homework: "We continue with these special moments at home and create new special moments."

Eia Asen pointed out that the therapist's role modelling as a very good parental figure is a key non-specific factor. He argued that it was important to discuss whether this role model function is a non-specific factor to be built into therapy. It is also important to consider and discuss when to transfer the responsibility to the parents, and at what point role modelling becomes too imposing on the parents, who might feel that they are not "good enough". He mentioned that it had occurred to him when he saw how Theraplay used soap bubbles, for example, and the parent who is observing might say, "Ah, I must try that as well." And, of course, the mother will not do it in the same way as the therapist, which is fine, but seeing this behaviour gives her permission to be playful, silly, and to engage in activities with her children that have no purpose besides being fun and enjoyable. The point is to see another adult, who is supposed to be doing serious therapeutic work, acting in this playful, silly manner. Jukka Mäkelä agreed, and added that it is important to explain to the parents, explicitly and unambiguously, that there are many different ways of being a good parent. Therefore, what the parent sees the therapist do with the child might look very different from what the parent does, yet both approaches can be equally good and valid. Thus, modelling is not about copying, but about picking up on the same elements.

Peter Levine said that just as therapy is about working with the child's zone of proximal development, having a good dialogue also requires working with the parents' zone of proximal development. We commented that another aspect of acting as a role model is that the child becomes important in the eyes of the parent when the child's skills and capacities are recognised. This relates to a different aspect of being a role model, which is that the parents should adopt this ability to acknowledge their child, even if they do it in a different way than the therapist; observing the interactions between the therapist and the child gives the parents an opportunity to grasp this. Haldor Øvreeide argued that supporting the parents' development first of all requires helping them to observe their child and his or her reactions. Thus, when he looks at what the parents do, the reflections always revolve around the question, "What is the child showing?" and "What do we see in the child?" Good automatic parenting is about reading the child accurately. If the therapist places too much emphasis on being a role model in the sense of showing the parents "this is what you should do", the parents will focus more on themselves than on the child. It is also important to help the child display a response that is interesting and relevant to the parent. Jukka Mäkelä commented that one of the key aspects of the therapist's functions as a role model is to focus on the moment. When the parents stop worrying about what is going on and, instead, just focus on the present moment, they can see what the child does, and how the child reacts. The role model function springs from seeing the child instead of merely understanding him or her on a cognitive level. It is the therapist's job to be silly, to be present in the moment, and to be observant, observing with curiosity who the child is, and share this awareness with the parents. As Haldor Øvreeide commented, the therapist should help the parents share the joy over the child. We commented that an essential point of the role model function is to operate on a limbic rather than a prefrontal level, because, if the process is prefrontal, there is a right and a wrong way for the parents to proceed and, thus, a risk of failure.

## Ensuring continuity outside the therapy room

Jukka Mäkelä explained that Theraplay involves assigning homework from session one. When the parents see the child enjoying a particular aspect of what is going on in the therapy session, the therapist or the parent considers how that moment might be recreated at home. Typically, the therapist suggests doing it in the evening, at bedtime. The therapist explains, "Nothing big; just do this one little thing and that's fine." Eia Asen added that at the Marlborough Family Service, when they do something in a session, they always consider how it might be generalised to the home or other situations, so that the learning or experiences can be exported to the home environment. This is often achieved by giving the parents homework in the form of tasks or assignments. This homework is always based on a specific experience or a now moment. Eia Asen mentioned that, over the years, he had seen many great assignments, his own included, that were simply too demanding and, therefore, were never carried out. For example, the Milan group (the founders of the Milan School of systemic family treatment method, the psychiatrists Gianfranco Cecchin, Luigi Boscolo, Mara Selvini Pallazzoli, and Giuliana Prata) formulated amazing assignments that no one ever did; at best, the parents pretended they had done them. Therefore, the homework assignments should always spring from the moment, an experience that can be replicated at home in a fun way. We rounded off by pointing out that this reflected a perfect transition from the child's developmental process to the parents' developmental process; this transition is important, since the parents have to be able to support and contain the child.

One of the conference participants commented that Haldor Øvreeide seems to insist on always having the carer present in the room. The person asked what are the most important or core reasons for that, and whether there would be cases when Haldor Øvreeide would choose to work just with the child. Haldor Øvreeide replied that he never allows an abusive parent into the therapy room. He said he also would not want to include parents who are too defensive. He said that he might include a carer who has subjected the child to some degree of neglect, but, in that case, he would work with the parent first, one-on-one. When working with children in a triadic context, he has to optimise his relationship with the parent, and if he has a problem in his relationship with the parent he has to re-establish that relationship before bringing in the child too much. The parent has to be receptive to the child, and Haldor Øvreeide has to trust that he will be able to make the parent receptive to the child. As a psychotherapist, he prefers to work with someone who is involved in caring for the child on a daily basis; someone who can carry the narrative from the session into the child's daily life. As Jukka Mäkelä pointed out, one of the key non-specific factors is to make sure that there is someone who can carry the structure into real life and preserve a degree of continuity.

Eia Asen added that at the Marlborough Family Service, to determine who should take part in the therapy, they usually start with a telephone call. They also use telephones in their sessions, just as Haldor Øvreeide did, but they use the telephone before the therapy has even begun, because today even the poorest families have mobile phones. In a tongue-in-cheek remark, Eia Asen said that, in his experience, some poor families use the little money they have to buy several mobile phones and plasma television screens rather than healthy foods.

In this initial phone call, they begin to establish the context in terms of who should take part. They might ask the person who takes the call, "We've got this case, it's been referred by the doctor (or the social services or the court or whatever)—who should come the first time?" They might say, "Maybe I should come." Then we say, "Well, what are the advantages and disadvantages of you coming on your own? What would happen if your husband came, and should the child be there?" Thus, the first session at the Marlborough Family Service is always preceded by some shared considerations and decision-making processes. They accept whoever comes in the first time, but continue to make and remake the person context, that is, who comes in for the given session, over and over again.

*Parents should be supported in trusting, taking responsibility, and being engaged in their ability to create positive changes for and with their child*

As Haldor Øvreeide described in his presentation at the conference, the child enters into the interactions with the parents with an intrinsic motivation for development, and there is no doubt about the child's will or engagement in the world. The child's intrinsic developmental competence must be met by relevant responses from carers to support the unfolding of the child's capacities. However, this is embedded in a cultural project. The cultural environment has an influence on the response that the parents give the child. The parents enter into the situation with a cultural project that they carry on their shoulders. Thus, there are two projects to be aware of when interacting with the child. For the therapist, it is essential to consider how these two projects relate to the child's development, and whether they interact to promote the child's development, or whether they are a source of conflict and stress. It is important to know how the parents perceive their role in raising the child in order to determine if the parents' principles and their understanding of their own role form a context that is capable of supporting the child's development.

Haldor Øvreeide referred to an example from his demonstration video with Olaf to explain the two projects. Before the session shown in the video, Olaf's mother had told Haldor Øvreeide that the child protection services had told her that Olaf could have no contact with the stepfather. However, Haldor Øvreeide did not think that this was an accurate representation of what the child protection services had actually said. He said that parents often cast themselves as victims of circumstance, thus relinquishing their responsibility for the child. In that case, it is essential to reinstate the parents in their role as responsible actors. The mother was not taking responsibility, so

Haldor Øvreeide chose to do so temporarily, acting as an advocate for the child. Reinstating the parents in a position of responsibility is crucial. In relation to this point, Haldor Øvreeide also referred to a book he co-authored with his wife and colleague, Reidun Hafstad, titled *Utviklingsstøtte* ("Developmental Support", 2011). In this book, among other topics, they discuss the key issue of power and how to reinstate parents in a position of responsibility. The therapist has to take a stand, but how one defends this position is crucial. For example, it is important not to become moralistic but, instead, to present moral challenges. In the clip with Olaf, we saw that the mother had collapsed mentally. Peter Levine added that when he saw the interaction between Olaf and the mother, for example, at the end when he put his ear to mother's heart, and when he sent the drawing to the stepfather, he saw a love connection that he thought was absolutely critical. He also said that he had wondered if it was a problem that, in a sense, the boy was giving away his heart to his parents; he gave his heart to his mother, who was depressed, anxious, and could not sleep, and to the stepfather, who was taking drugs. Haldor Øvreeide agreed with Peter Levine's assessment that Olaf responded to a difficult situation by taking emotional care of the parents in order to preserve the relationship. If he had continued to care for his parents like this, he would have been exhausted. However, he was trying to keep his family together, and, in that sense, he was fighting for his own life. This was evident, for example, when he brought in the juice bottle, saying "Mummy!" in a deliberately cheerful and appealing tone. Here, he was trying to lift the emotional situation. He often looked at his mother and seemed to be preoccupied with "How is my mother reacting?" Haldor Øvreeide explained that he had previously worked with the mother in therapy, and after the session in the video, he followed up on that intervention.

## Working with multi-generation families

Family therapy often involves a large group of people, and it is important to identify the family members who can best support the child. As Eia Asen pointed out, the therapist has to consider when to pass on the baton. At the Marlborough Family Service, for example, they consider when they can pass on the baton to the father or the mother, and the therapist can leave the room. Most of their cases are finished in six or eight sessions. Peter Levine commented that this reminded him of a woman he had worked with many years ago. She had been completely debilitated since an experience in her early twenties when she was visiting her boyfriend, now husband. This was in New England in the autumn, and the leaves were turning colour. She met a hunter in the woods, and he took his rifle and hit her in the head. She fell to the ground, and he kept hitting her over and over again. Afterwards, she was suffering from severe symptoms of depression, dysfunction, and anxiety. In the sessions with Peter Levine she made excellent progress. But then she got to a point where after the session she would be really fine, and then she would bang her head on something, a drawer in the kitchen or a mirror in the bathroom, one thing or another. Around the same time, Peter Levine was also working with her son, who was an elite athlete and had been in an accident. Eventually, Peter Levine had her bring her family together, three generations. Simply sitting together and telling their stories helped to eliminate the repetitions of the original traumas, but as long as he was working with the woman alone, he was unable to get to that point. In connection with this discussion, Jukka Mäkelä mentioned Sarah Hrdy's research; she documented that some 100 years ago, a child would be surrounded by a group of about 150 people, and points out the importance of the groups around the family. For a young child, the relationship with a single person might seem to be of overwhelming importance, but later, there are many people to support the child.

## Supporting the professional network around the child

Jukka Mäkelä mentioned that the idea is not to have the therapist alone provide children with developmentally supportive experiences; the therapist should prepare not only the parents, but also preschool teachers, teachers, and nurses to provide these experiences when they are with the children to ensure that the child has access to healthy experiences through all the adults in his or her life.

Waqar, who, in many regards, is similar to Matias, was in a foster family, and the foster mother had difficulty handling him. He was wild, out of control, and acted aggressively towards the other children in his preschool class. The foster mother had to come and get him from school, not every week, but every day, because the teachers could not control his aggressive behaviour and he refused to accept orders. Essentially, Waqar was terrified, and this was an important understanding to convey both to his foster parents and to the preschool teachers and other adults in his life. There was a general consensus that therapy is not just about supporting the child in the therapy room and in interactions with the parents; it is also about ensuring that the child is supported in interactions with significant others, for example, by providing supervision to key professionals in the child's life.

## *Summary*

At the conference, all four psychotherapists agreed that therapy with children requires inclusion of the parents and the rest of the family as well as the everyday network around the child. In addition to the carer's crucial influence on the child's personality development, it is also important how the other family members relate to each other, including the relationship with grandparents and the parents' siblings. In current western culture, children are influenced by a wide range of relational experiences, including preschool, school, and peer groups, but the relationship between carer and child and the family unit in general are still the venue of the child's attachment and their primary source of care.

In any therapy context, it is important to support the carers in their responsibility and to give them the space to be active and responsible participants in what needs to happen to alleviate their child's difficulties. Child therapists are not authority figures who hold the solution to the parents' difficulties, but they can take a curious and explorative stance in interactions with the child and experiment with more satisfying ways of being together. The condition for a successful therapeutic process is that the parents receive help to discover their own potential, to have faith in their parental behaviour, and to be curious about themselves and the child. It is important to appeal to the parents' curiosity and to reinstate them as authority figures in their life with the child. The therapist must attempt to reach and activate the parents' emotional and mental capacity, and in this process the parents' mental processing plays a crucial role.

The family therapy process draws the parents' attention to aspects and expressions in their child that they had not previously noticed. It is important to try to help the parents generate more reality-adapted representations of the child and act in accordance with them; this is done in part by confronting the carer with the real child as the therapist sees him or her.

At the conference, Øvreeide pointed out, as he has also done repeatedly in his books, that the dialogue between a therapist and a child is a dyadic process with triadic consequences. Thus, by entering into a therapy process with a child, the therapist gives the child an opportunity to be seen and contained with his or her difficulties, and he or she also gives the parents an opportunity to see their child in a new light. The therapist attempts to engage in attunement and in a dialogue with the child that the parents have failed to establish, because the child's difficulties often stem from the parents' failure to attune properly with the child's needs and problems.

Thus, from the beginning of the conversation, the therapist should take the lead in order to challenge the child's maladaptive relational pattern, but, as soon as possible, the responsibility should be transferred to the parents, where it belongs. At first, the parents might lean on the therapist and use him or her as a role model for attending to and interacting with the child. As a role model, the therapist should help to make the child significant in the eyes of the parents. By observing the child's interactions with the therapist, the parents should come to experience and understand their child in a new light and, thus, learn to acknowledge the child. Just as therapy should take place in the child's zone of proximal development, it should also address the parents' zone of proximal development in order to establish a productive dialogue.

# CHAPTER TWELVE

# Closing remarks

"In working with these kids we have to forge a strong connection where they can feel validated as strong individuals and
not fragile plants"

(Eia Asen)

Over the years, many researchers have pointed out the crucial
importance of early relations for the development of
emotional, personal, and social capacities and described how
attunement processes in this early period come to light in the therapist–client relationship later in life. After millions of years of evolution, the human brain is now "designed" to be able to synchronise
with other people's nervous systems. All therapy systems include a
large number of non-specific factors that play a key role in generating
change processes, but which the therapist does not necessarily focus
on or consider important. As long as the method works, of course, we
need not worry about these factors. However, if we wish to continue
to develop useful and varied services, we will need to identify these
non-specific factors, and that requires a significant research effort. The
purpose of the two-day conference and this book, *Through Windows of*

*Opportunity*, has been to take some initial steps towards identifying these factors.

The human motivation to establish emotional attachments is innate, and the change in the psychotherapeutic relationship takes place through microscopic moments of meeting, which lead to equally microscopic changes in the neural circuits. In connection with personality development, the stimulation takes place through dyadic processes, and, in therapy with children, it takes place ideally in triadic processes, as the parents play an absolutely critical role in supporting the child in his or her psychological development processes. The therapy process gives the child novel experiences; they do not repair the past, but build a new inner representation that can be integrated in the nervous system. The changes to the neural circuits make it possible to establish a new context where more new experiences can emerge. The therapy process, with its many present moments, makes it possible to rewrite old history and to develop more adaptive relational patterns between child and parents. We develop our emotional skills by living life in the present in the framework of human interactions; this leads to learning that takes place deep inside our procedural memory, long before the content aspect of language comes into play. Stern (2004) has pointed out repeatedly that events must be lived, with feelings and actions taking place in real time, in the real world, with real people.

Perhaps the most important outcomes of psychotherapy with children are emotional tolerance between child and parents, affect regulation, and the development of, especially, the parents' mentalization capacities, because this process enables the child to engage in synchronised attunement processes with others and, thus, secure psychological development processes and the capacity for self-regulation. Therapy involves many objectives and milestones in the maturation hierarchy and neural reorganisation. Therapy is about establishing attachment and relationships, but also about building mentalization capacity. It is about challenging fixated patterns and generating an integration process within the child's and, not least, the parents', zones of proximal development. Profound transformation processes are driven by the fundamental human need to feel seen and understood by others. In evolutionary terms, this need arose from the basic mammalian need to feel socially connected with others. The goal of the therapy process is to establish the mutual emotional attunement between child and parents, and to achieve this, the therapist has to act as "the magical stranger" who is present for a while to help set the process in motion. The only thing that can heal inadequate attachment is the establishing of an attachment that is based on adaptive emotional attunement.

In closing, we once again give the floor to the four psychotherapists who made this conference possible, Peter Levine, Jukka Mäkelä, Haldor Øvreeide, and Eia Asen, and share with you some of the words they used to summarise the conference:

Peter Levine suggested that the participants use their dorsolateral prefrontal cortices to relate the themes of the conference to their pre-existing schemas, considering how they fit, and which parts are consonant, which are dissonant, and which parts they might want to think more about. The conference took at look at the non-specific data in apparently very diverse systems, as factors that are not tied into "your method", "my method", but as something that is much more general or underneath. Peter Levine's suggestion to the audience was, "As you leave today and take a walk in the beautiful Copenhagen summer, which is almost here, start to just shift a little bit, to just kind of let this stuff slosh around inside of yourselves, and pick some things that maybe informed or inspired you, or confused you, and to write down your dreams and just to notice how these things take root in your fertile soils."

Jukka Mäkelä said that he was very happy that the publisher of the Danish book, Hans Reitzels, had hired someone to take notes to make it possible to organise in written form the non-specific factors that we have been collecting or touching on: in his mind, he said, they were all still in a blur. He mentioned that one of the concepts he had found stimulating was the concept of advocacy. Naturally, as therapists, they had all been taught that moments of meeting, real relationships, etc., are important non-specific factors, but now there was also talk of magic and things like that! He said that he was still a little confused, so he thought that Peter Levine's idea of *sloshing* was a good example of what was going to happen in his mind!

Haldor Øvreeide said that he was happy that his wife and colleague, Reidun Hafstad, was here with him, so that he could discuss the events of the day with her. He was hoping that many of the participants also had colleagues with whom to continue the discussion. He said that it was important to share experiences, thoughts, etc., and, for him, the conference had been a great opportunity to share thoughts, listen to the others—in fact, he felt the event had been developmentally supportive for him! In closing, he reminded everyone that the experience is always stored in the individual—we find it in ourselves, not in others.

Eia Asen said that he had written seventeen pages of notes from the conference, which were now in his computer. He said that it had been two fantastic days, probably as much for the presenters as for the audience. Because all the therapists present work in very different working contexts, and often also in different cultures, and because different working contexts bring forth different methods and different ideas, he thought it had been a good feature to have presenters from different countries. This added to the richness, because the presenters worked in different contexts and saw very different types of clients. He considered any form of therapy that only offers one answer to all problems depressing to see, and was delighted to note that the two-day conference had been quite the opposite of that.

For us, it has been a pleasure to edit this book about the experiences from the conference. Many important points were highlighted, and we have now had a chance to digest and organise some of the highlights in these chapters. As many of the points followed close on each other's heels at the conference, it has been a rewarding experience to spend some time considering the many reflections that the four presenters shared with us. We hope that anyone who reads this book, both the participants who were present at the conference and others who share, will find some measure of the inspiration that we found in both the two-day event and the editing process.

# REFERENCES

Aitken, K. J., & Trevarthen, C. (1997). Self–other organization in human psychological development. *Development and Psychopathology, 9*: 651–675.

Ammaniti, M., & Gallese, V. (Eds.) (2014). *The Birth of Intersubjectivity: Psychodynamics, Neurobiology, and the Self.* New York: Norton.

Asen, E. (2005). Connecting systems and psyche. Psyche and systems: the inner world—the outer world. Conference, LO-skolen, 9 March 2005.

Beebe, B., & Lachmann, F. M. (2002). *Infant Research and Adult Treatment: Co-Constructing Interactions.* Hillsdale, NJ: Analytic Press.

Bentzen, M., & Hart, S. (2012). Jegets fundament: Den neuroaffektive udviklings første vækstbølge og de neuroaffektive kompasser. In: S. Hart (Ed.), *Neuroaffektiv psykoterapi med voksne* (pp. 105–148). Copenhagen: Hans Reitzels.

Bentzen, M., & Hart, S. (2013). Empati, dynamik og læringsperspektiver i lederens personlighedsudvikling. In: S. Hart & H. Hvilshøj (Eds.), *Ledelse mellem hjerne og hjerte* (pp. 55–95). Copenhagen: Hans Reitzels.

Bion, W. R. (1962). *Learning from Experience.* New York: Basic Books.

Booth, P. B., & Jernberg, A. M. (2009). *Theraplay: Helping Parents and Children Build Better Relationships through Attachment-Based Play* (3rd edn). San Francisco: Jossey-Bass.

Bowlby, J. (1988). *A Secure Base: Clinical Applications of Attachment Theory.* London: Routledge.

Bowlby, J. (1991). The role of the psychotherapist's personal resources in the therapeutic situation. *Bulletin of the British Psychoanalytic Society,* 27(11): 26–30.

Bråten, S. (1993). The virtual other in infants' minds and social feelings. In: A. H. Wold (Ed.), *The Dialogical Alternative* (pp. 77–97). Oslo: Scandinavian University Press.

Bråten, S. (1998). *Kommunikasjon og samspill fra fødsel til alderdom.* Oslo: Scandinavian University Press.

Brazelton, T. B., & Cramer, B. G. (1990). *The Earliest Relationship: Parents, Infants, and the Drama of Early Attachment.* Cambridge: Perseus Books.

Bruner, J. S. (1985). Vygotsky: a historical and conceptual perspective. In: J. Wertsch (Ed.), *Culture, Communication and Cognition: Vygotskian Perspectives* (pp. 21–34). Cambridge: Cambridge University Press.

Bruner, J. S. (1990). *Acts of Meaning.* Cambridge, MA: Harvard University Press.

Chamley, C. A., Carson, P., & Randall, D. (2005). *Developmental Anatomy and Physiology of Children: A Practical Approach.* London: Churchill Livingstone.

Chugani, H. T., & Phelps, M. E. (1986). Maturational changes in cerebral function in infants determined by FDG position emission tomography. *Science, 231*(4740): 840–843.

Chugani, H. T., Phelps, M. E., & Mazziotta, J. C. (1987). Position emission tomography: study of human brain functional development. *Annals of Neurology, 22*(4): 487–497.

Cicchetti, D., & Tucker, D. (1994). Development and self-regulation structures of the mind. *Development and Psychopathology, 6*(4): 533–549.

Cozolino, L. J. (2002). *The Neuroscience of Psychotherapy: Building and Rebuilding the Human Brain.* New York: Norton.

Damasio, A. R. (1999). *The Feeling of What Happens: Body, Emotion and the Making of Consciousness.* New York: Harcourt Brace.

Donaldson, M. (1978). *Children's Minds.* Glasgow: Fontana/Collins.

Dunn, J. (1996). The Emanuel Miller Memorial Lecture 1995: Children's relationships—bridging the divide between cognitive and social development. *Journal of Child Psychology and Psychiatry, 37*(5): 507–518.

Eckerdal, P., & Merker, B. (2009). 'Music' and the 'action song' in infant development: an interpretation. In: S. Malloch & C. Trevarthen (Eds.), *Communicative Musicality: Exploring the Basis of Human Companionship* (pp. 241–262). Oxford: Oxford University Press.

Emde, R. N. (1989). The infant's relationship experience: developmental and affective aspects. In: J. Sameroff & R. N. Emde (Eds.), *Relationship Disturbances in Early Childhood: A Developmental Approach* (pp. 33–51). New York: Basic Books.

Emde, R. N. (1992). Social referencing: uncertainty, self and the search for meaning. In: S. Feinman (Ed.), *Social Referencing and the Social Construction of Reality in Infancy* (pp. 79–94). London: Plenum Press.

Fair, D. A., Cohen, A. L., Power, J. D., Dosenbach, N. U. F., Church, J. A., Miezin, F. M., Schlaggar, B. L., & Petersen, S. E. (2009). Functional brain networks develop from a "local to distributed" organization. *PLoS Computational Biology, 5*(5): e1000381.

Fonagy, P. (1998). Moments of change in psychoanalytic theory: discussion of a new theory of psychic change. *Infant Mental Health Journal, 19*(3): 346–353.

Fonagy, P. (1999). Memory and therapeutic action. *International Journal of Psychoanalysis, 80*: 215–223.

Fonagy, P. (2005). Connecting the intrapsychic and the interpersonal. Psyche and systems: the inner world—the outer world. Conference, LO-skolen, 9 March 2005.

Fonagy, P., Gergely, G., Jurist, E. L., & Target, M. (2007). *Affektregulering, mentalisering og selvets udvikling.* Copenhagen: Akademisk.

Fonagy, P., Target, M., & Gergely, G. (2000). Attachment and borderline personality disorder: a theory and some evidence. *Psychiatric Clinics of North America, 23*(1): 103–122.

Freeman, W. (1995). *Societies of Brains: A Study in the Neuroscience of Love and Hate.* Hillsdale, NJ: Lawrence Erlbaum.

Frønes, I. (1994). *De ligeværdige: Om socialisering og de jævnaldrendes betydning.* Copenhagen: Børn & Unge.

Gerhardt, S. (2004). *Why Love Matters: How Affection Shapes a Baby's Brain.* New York: Brunner-Routledge.

Gjærum, B., & Ellertsen, B. (2002). *Hjerne og atferd: Utviklingsforstyrrelser hos barn og ungdom i et nevrobiologisk perspektiv.* Oslo: Gyldendal.

Goldberg, E. (2001). *The Executive Brain: Frontal Lobes and the Civilized Mind.* New York: Oxford University Press.

Goleman, D. (2003). *Destructive Emotions. How Can We Overcome Them? A Scientific Dialogue with the Dalai Lama.* New York: Bantam Books.

Goodrich, B. G. (2010). We do, therefore we think: time, motility, and consciousness. *Reviews in the Neurosciences, 21*(5): 331–361.

Gunnar, M., & Vazquez, D. (2001). Social regulation of the cortisol levels in early human development. *Psychoneuroendocrinology, 27*: s. 199–220.

Hafstad, R., & Øvreeide, H. (2007). Det tredje ansikt i barnets relasjoner. In: H. Haavind & H. Øvreeide (Eds.), *Barn og unge i psykoterapi: Samspill og utviklingsforståelse* (pp. 97–137). Oslo: Gyldendal Akademisk.

Hammer, E. (1990). *Reaching the Affect: Style in the Psychodynamic Therapies.* London: Jason Aronson.

Hart, S. (2008). *Brain, Attachment, Personality: An Introduction to Neuro-affective Development.* London: Karnac.

Hart, S. (2009). *Den følsomme hjerne: Hjernens udvikling gennem tilknytning og samhørighedsbånd.* Copenhagen: Hans Reitzels.

Hart, S. (2010). *The Impact of Attachment.* New York: Norton.

Hart, S. (Ed.) (2011). *Neuroaffektiv psykoterapi med børn.* Copenhagen: Hans Reitzels.

Hart, S. (Ed.) (2012). *Neuroaffektiv psykoterapi med voksne.* Copenhagen: Hans Reitzels.

Hart, S., & Kæreby, F. (2012). Dialogen med det autonome nervesystem i den psykoterapeutiske proces: at støtte resiliens og afhjælpe traumatisk stress i lyset af arousalregulering. In: S. Hart, S. (Ed.), *Neuroaffektiv psykoterapi med voksne* (pp. 243–264). Copenhagen: Hans Reitzels.

Hart, S., & Schwartz, R. (2008). *Fra interaktion til relation: Tilknytning hos Winnicott, Bowlby, Stern, Schore & Fonagy.* Copenhagen: Hans Reitzels.

Hobson, R. P. (1993). The emotional origins of social understanding. *Philosophical Psychology, 6*(3): 227–249.

Hubel, D. H., & Wiesel, T. N. (1970). The period of susceptibility to the physiological effects of unilateral eye closure in kittens. *Journal of Physiology, 206*(2): 419–436.

Jackson, J. H. (1958). *Selected Writings of John Hughlings Jackson: Evolution and Dissolution of the Nervous System, Speech, Various Papers, Addresses, and Lectures.* London: Stables.

Karr-Morse, R., & Wiley, M. (1997). *Ghosts from the Nursery: Tracing the Roots of Violence.* New York: Atlantic Monthly Press.

Kugiumutzakis, G., & Trevarthen, C. (2014). Neonatal imitation. In: J. Wright (Ed.), *The International Encyclopedia of the Social and Behavioral Sciences* (2nd edn). Oxford: Elsevier.

Levine, P. (1983). Chronic perinatal stress as a predisposing factor in autism and childhood psychosis: a neurodevelopmental model suggesting strategies in treatment and prophylaxis. Paper presented to Symposium on Autism. Montreal/San Francisco: University du Quebec a Montreal/San Francisco State University.

Levine, P., & Kline, M. (2006). *Trauma through a Child's Eyes: Awakening the Ordinary Miracle of Healing*. Berkeley, CA: North Atlantic Books.

Levine, P., & Kline, M. (2009). *Trauma Proofing Your Kids: A Parent's Guide for Instilling Confidence, Joy, and Resilience*. Berkeley, CA: North Atlantic Books.

Levy, D. (1945). Psychic trauma of operations in children and a note on combat neurosis. *American Journal of Diseases of Children, 69*: 7–25.

Lewis, T., Amini, F., & Lannon, R. (2001). *A General Theory of Love*. New York: Vintage Books.

Lyons-Ruth, K. (1998). Implicit relational knowing: its role in development and psychoanalytic treatment. *International Mental Health Journal, 19*(3): 282–289.

MacLean, P. D. (1990). *The Triune Brain in Evolution: Role in Paleocerebral Functions*. New York: Plenum Press.

Morgan, A. (1998). Moving along to things left undone. *Infant Mental Health Journal, 19*(3): 324–332.

Neisser, U. (1993). The self perceived. In: U. Neisser (Ed.), *The Perceived Self: Ecological and Interpersonal Sources of Self Knowledge* (pp. 3–21). New York: Cambridge University Press.

Orlinsky, D. E., & Howard, K. I. (1986). Process and outcome in psychotherapy. In: S. L. Garfield & A. E. Bergin (Eds.), *Handbook of Psychotherapy and Behaviour Change* (pp. 311–384). New York: Wiley.

Øvreeide, H. (2001). Barnet som familieterapeutisk bruker. *Fokus på familien, 29*(1): 22–35.

Øvreeide, H. (2002). *Samtaler med barn: Metodiske samtaler med barn i vanskelige livssituasjoner*. Kristiansand: Høyskoleforlaget.

Øvreeide, H., & Hafstad, R. (2011). *Utviklingsstøtte: Foreldrefokusert arbeid med barn*. Kristiansand: CappelenDamm Høyskoleforlaget.

Panksepp, J. (1998). *Affective Neuroscience. The Foundations of Human and Animal Emotions*. New York: Oxford University Press.

Panksepp, J., & Biven, L. (2012). *The Archaeology of Mind: Neuroevolutionary Origins of Human Emotions*. New York: Norton.

Perry, B. (2002). Childhood experience and the expression of genetical potential: what childhood neglect tells us about nature and nurture. *Brain and Mind, 3*(1): 79–100.

Porges, S. W. (1995). Orienting in a defensive world: mammalian modifications of our evolutionary heritage: a polyvagal theory. *Psychophysiology, 32*(4): 301–318.

Porges, S. W. (1997). Emotion: an evolutionary by-product of the neural regulation of the autonomic nervous system. In: C. S. Carter,

B. Kirkpatrick, & I. I. Lederhendler (Eds.), *The Integrative Neurobiology of Affiliation*. New York: New York Academy of Sciences.

Porges, S. W. (1998). Love: an emergent property of the mammalian autonomic nervous system. *Psychoneuroendocrinology*, 23(8): 837–861.

Porges, S. W. (2003). Social engagement and attachment: a phylogenetic perspective. Roots of mental illness in children. *Annals of the New York Academy of Sciences*, *1008*: 31–47.

Rizzolatti, G., & Arbib, M. (1998). Language within our grasp. *Trends in Neurosciences*, 21(5): 188–194.

Roth, A., & Fonagy, P. (1996). *What Works for Whom? A Critical Review of Psychotherapy Research* (2nd edn). New York: Guilford Press.

Rutter, M., & Rutter, M. (1997). *Den livslange udvikling*. Copenhagen: Hans Reitzels.

Sameroff, A. (1989). Principles of development and psychopathology. In: J. Sameroff & R. N. Emde (Eds.), *Relationship Disturbances in Early Childhood: A Developmental Approach* (pp. 297–312). New York: Basic Books.

Sander, L. W. (1977). The regulation of exchange in the infant-caregiver system and some aspects of the context-content relationship. In: M. Lewis & L. A. Rosenblum (Eds.), *Interaction, Conversation, and the Development of Language* (pp. 133–155). New York: John Wiley.

Sander, L. W. (1983). Polarity, paradox, and the organizing process in development. In: J. D. Call, E. Galenson, & R. L. Tyson (Eds.), *Frontiers of Infant Psychiatry, 1* (pp. 333–347). New York: Basic Books.

Sander, L. W. (1988). The event structure of regulation in the neonate–caregiver system as a biological background for early organization of psychic structure. In: A. Goldberg (Ed.) *Frontiers in Self Psychology, 3* (pp. 3–27). Hillsdale, NJ: Analytic Press.

Sander, L. W. (1992). Letter to the Editor. *International Journal of Psychoanalysis*, 73: 582–584.

Sander, L. W. (1995). Thinking about developmental process: wholeness, specificity, and the organization of conscious experiencing. Speech at the annual meeting in the Division of Psychoanalysis, American Psychological Association, Santa Monica, April 1995.

Schibbye, A. L. L. (2005). *Relationer: Et dialektisk perspektiv*. Copenhagen: Akademisk.

Schore, A. N. (1994). *Affect Regulation and the Origin of Self*. Hillsdale, NJ: Lawrence Erlbaum.

Schore, A. N. (2003a). *Affect Dysregulation and Disorders of the Self*. New York: Norton.

Schore, A. N. (2003b). *Affect Regulation and the Repair of the Self*. New York: Norton.

Siegel, D. J. (1999). *The Developing Mind: Toward a Neurobiology of Interpersonal Experience*. New York: Guilford Press.

Spitz, R. (1952). *Psychogenic Diseases in Infancy. Psychoanalytic Research Project on Problems of Infancy* (film).

Sroufe, L. A. (1979). Socioemotional development. In: J. Osofsky (Ed.), *Handbook of Infant Development* (pp. 462–516). New York: Wiley.

Sroufe, L. A. (1989). Relationships, self, and individual adaptation. In: J. Sameroff & R. N. Emde (Eds.), *Relationship Disturbances in Early Childhood: A Developmental Approach* (pp. 70–94). New York: Basic Books.

Sroufe, L. A. (1996). *Emotional Development: The Organization of Emotional Life in the Early Years*. New York: Cambridge University Press.

Stern, D. N. (1977). *The First Relationship: Infant and Mother*. Cambridge: Harvard University Press.

Stern, D. N. (1984). Affect attunement. In: J. D. Call, E. Galenson, & R. L. Tyson (Eds.), *Frontiers of Infant Psychiatry*, 2 (pp. 3–14). New York: Basic Books.

Stern, D. N. (1985). *The Interpersonal World of the Infant: A View from Psychoanalysis and Developmental Psychology*. New York: Basic Books.

Stern, D. N. (1990). Joy and satisfaction in infancy. In: R. A. Glick & S. Bone (Eds.), *Pleasure Beyond the Pleasure Principle* (pp. 13–25). New Haven, CT: Yale University Press.

Stern, D. N. (1995). *The Motherhood Constellation*. New York: Basic Books.

Stern, D. N. (1998a). The process of therapeutic change involving implicit knowledge: some implications of developmental observations for adult psychotherapy. *Infant Mental Health Journal*, 19(3): 300–308.

Stern, D. N. (1998b). Seminar and workshop, DISPUK, Snekkersten, 18–19 June 1998.

Stern, D. N. (2001). Lecture at the SICON conference, 9 November 2001, Copenhagen.

Stern, D. N. (2004). *The Present Moment in Psychotherapy and Everyday Life*. New York: Norton.

Stern, D. N., Sander, L. W., Nahum, J. P., Harrison, A. M., Lyons-Ruth, K., Morgan, A. C., Bruschweiler-Stern, N., & Tronick, E. Z. (1998). Non interpretive mechanisms in psychoanalytic therapy. *International Journal of Psychoanalysis*, 79: 903–921.

Supekar, K., Musen, M., & Menon, V. (2009). Development of large-scale functional brain networks in children. *PLoS Biology*, 7(7): e1000157.

Takada, A. (2005). Mother–infant interactions among the !Xun: analysis of gymnastic and breastfeeding behaviors. In: B. S. Hewlett & M. E. Lamb (Eds.), *Hunter-Gatherer Childhoods: Evolutionary, Developmental, and Cultural Perspectives* (pp. 289–308). New Brunswick, NJ: Aldine Transaction.

Tetzchner, S. (2002). *Utviklingspsykologi: Barne- og ungdomsalderen*. Oslo: Gyldendal Akademisk.

Thelen, E. (1989). Self-organization in developmental processes: can systems approaches work? In: M. Gunnar & E. Thelen (Eds.), *Systems and Development: The Minnesota Symposium in Child Psychology* (Vol. 22) (pp. 77–117). Hillsdale, NJ: Lawrence Erlbaum.

Thelen, E., & Smith, L. (1994). *A Dynamic Systems Approach to the Development of Cognition and Action*. Cambridge, MA: MIT Press.

Thormann, I., & Poulsen, I. (2013). *Spædbarnsterapi i behandling af et traumatiseret barn*. Copenhagen: Hans Reitzels.

Trevarthen, C. (1979). Communication and cooperation in early infancy: a description of primary intersubjectivity. In: M. Bullowa (Ed.), *Before Speech: The Beginning of Interpersonal Communication* (pp. 321–348). Cambridge: Cambridge University Press.

Trevarthen, C. (1986). Development of intersubjective motor control in infants. In: M. G. Wade & H. T. A. Whiting (Eds.), *Motor Development In Children: Aspects of Coordination and Control* (pp. 227–270). Dordrecht, Martinus Nijhof.

Trevarthen, C. (1990). Growth and education of the hemispheres. In: C. Trevarthen (Ed.), *Brain Circuits and Functions of the Mind* (pp. 334–363). Cambridge: Cambridge University Press.

Trevarthen, C. (1993a). The function of emotions in early infant communication and development. In: J. Nadel & L. Camaioni (Eds.), *New Perspectives in Early Communicative Development* (pp. 48–81). London: Routledge.

Trevarthen, C. (1993b). The self born in intersubjectivity: the psychology of an infant communicating. In: U. Neisser (Ed.), *The Perceived Self: Ecological and Interpersonal Sources of Self Knowledge* (pp. 121–173). New York: Cambridge University Press.

Trevarthen, C. (2006). First things first: infants make good use of the sympathetic rhythm of imitation, without reason or language. *Journal of Child Psychotherapy*, 31(1): 91–113.

Trevarthen, C., & Aitken, K. J. (2003). Regulation of brain development and age-related changes in infants' motives: the developmental function of "regressive" periods. In: M. Heimann (Ed.), *Regression*

*Periods in Human Infancy* (pp. 107–184). Mahwah, NJ: Lawrence Erlbaum.

Trevarthen, C., & Delafield-Butt, J. (2013). Biology of shared experience and language development: regulations for the inter-subjective life of narratives. In: M. Legerstee, D. Haley, & M. Bornstein (Eds.), *The Infant Mind: Origins of the Social Brain* (pp. 167–199). New York: Guildford Press.

Trevarthen, C., Aitken, K. J., Vandekerckhove, M., Delafield-Butt, J., & Nagy, E. (2006). Collaborative regulations of vitality in early childhood: stress in intimate relationships and postnatal psychopathology. In: D. Cicchetti & D. J. Cohen (Eds.), *Developmental Psychopathology, Volume 2, Developmental Neuroscience* (2nd edn) (pp. 65–126). New York: Wiley.

Uvnäs-Moberg, K. (1997a). Oxytocin linked antistress effects—the relaxation and growth response. *Acta Psychologica Scandinavica* (Suppl.), *640*: 38–42.

Uvnäs-Moberg, K. (1997b). Psychological and endocrine effects of social contact. In: C. S. Carter, I. I. Leder-Hendler, & B. Kirkpatrick (Eds.), *The Integrative Neurobiology of Affiliation. New York Academy of Sciences Annals*, *807*: 146–163.

Uvnäs-Moberg, K. (1998). Oxytocin may still mediate the benefits of positive social interaction and emotions. *Psychoneuroendocrinology*, *23*: 819–835.

Van der Kolk, B. A. (1987). *Psychological Trauma*. Washington: American Psychiatric Press.

Van der Kolk, B. A. (2000). Seminar in Sorø, Denmark, 3 July 2000.

Van der Kolk, B. A., & McFarlane, A. C. (1996). The black hole of trauma. In: B. A. van der Kolk, A. C. McFarlane, & L. Weisaeth (Eds.), *Traumatic Stress: The Effects of Overwhelming Experience on Mind, Body and Society*. New York: Guilford Press.

Vygotsky, L. S. (1978). *Mind in Society: The Development of Higher Psychological Processes*. Cambridge, MA: Harvard University Press.

Wampold, B. E. (2001). *The Great Psychotherapy Debate: Models, Methods, and Findings*. Mahwah, NJ: Lawrence Erlbaum.

Winnicott, D. W. (1960). The theory of the parent–infant relationship. *Journal of Psychoanalysis*, *41*: 585–595.

Winnicott, D. W. (1967). Mirror-role of mother and family in child development. In: *Playing and Reality* (pp. 111–118). London: Tavistock.

Winnicott, D. W. (1971). *Therapeutic Consultations in Child-Psychiatry*. New York: Basic Books.

# INDEX